The Book on Pregnancy After Loss:

The Exact Life-Changing Tools, Techniques, and Supplements I Used to Go From Losing 5 Babies to Safely Delivering 3 Healthy Babies All in Less Than 3.5 Years with Ease and Confidence

By: Tiphanie Jamison VanDerLugt, Esq.

The Yay Me University
ISBN-13: 978-1481879835
ISBN-10: 1481879839

For print or media interviews with Tiphanie please contact:
Press@TheYayMeUniversity.com

Tiphanie Jamison VanDerLugt
Telephone: 1 (760) 565-3106
Email: *Tiphanie@TheYayMeUniversity.com*

Limits of Liability and Disclaimer of Warranty:

endorsement of any website or sources. This book is sold with the express understanding that the author and publisher are not rendering medical, health, or personal services. The author and publisher disclaim all liability associated with the recommendations and guidelines set forth in this book.

The products and information (individually and collectively "The Materials") obtained through this website, including but not limited to personal consultations and from The Yay Me University, are for informational purposes only and are not intended to replace or substitute any advice from your medical practitioner, a qualified doctor, or any other professional and advisor. You should consult a qualified health practitioner before implementing any of the suggestions found on The Website, and should not give up any medical treatment you are using without the express consent of a medical professional.

The Materials obtained through The Website cannot serve as a substitute for face-to-face professional advice and are not intended to diagnose or treat any illness, metabolic disorder, disease or health problem. Always consult your physician or health care provider before beginning any nutrition or exercise program or using The Materials obtained through The Website. You voluntarily undertake your use of The Materials contained on The Website, and you assume all risk and responsibility for any such use, including but not limited to any increase in severity of your infertility condition. The Materials found on The Website may not be suitable for your own personal circumstances, you may not receive any benefit from use of The Materials, and The Website does not guarantee that you will achieve any specific result.

The Website is neither responsible nor liable for injury resulting from the use, misuse, and/or abuse of The Materials. You hereby release and agree to hold harmless The Website, its directors, officers, employees, agents, representatives, successors, advisors, consultants, and assigns from any and all causes of action and claims of any nature resulting from your use of The Materials.

The content and information accessed through The Website represents the content and information as at the date of publication. As conditions change, The Website reserves the right to alter and update the content to reflect the new conditions.

The Website does not assume any responsibility for errors, inaccuracies or omissions in any of the articles or information posted on the website. The website content may contain inaccuracies or typographical errors. This website may contain certain historical information. Historical information necessarily is not current and is provided for your reference only. Further, The Website is not responsible if information that is made available on this website is not accurate, reliable, complete, timely, or current. Any reliance upon the material on this website will be at your own risk. The Website reserves the right to modify the contents of the website at any time, but The Website has no obligation to update any information on this website. You agree that it is your responsibility to monitor changes to the website.

Tiphanie Jamison VanDerLugt, TheRadicalSelfExpert.com, The RADICAL Self ExpertMethod.com, TheBookonPregnancyAfterLoss.com, and any and all sites related to, owned and/or administrated by, including but not limited to ITS OWNERS, ITS AFFILIATES, AND ITS SPONSORS ARE NEITHER RESPONSIBLE NOR LIABLE FOR ANY DIRECT, INDIRECT, INCIDENTAL, CONSEQUENTIAL, SPECIAL, EXEMPLARY, PUNITIVE OR OTHER DAMAGES ARISING OUT OF OR RELATING IN ANY WAY TO THE SITE, SITE-RELATED SERVICES AND/OR CONTENT OR INFORMATION CONTAINED WITHIN THE SITE. YOUR SOLE REMEDY FOR DISSATISFACTION WITH THE SITE AND/OR SITE-RELATED SERVICES IS TO STOP USING THE SITE AND/OR THOSE SERVICES.

Disclaimer: The information on The Book on Pregnancy After Loss and all associated sites with Tiphanie, Jamison VanDerLugt is provided for educational purposes only and is not intended to treat, diagnose or prevent any disease. The entire contents of this website are based upon the opinions of Tiphanie Jamison VanDerLugt, unless otherwise noted. Individual articles are based upon the opinions of the respective author, who retains copyright as marked. The information on this website is not intended to replace a one-on-one relationship with a qualified health care professional and is not intended as medical advice. It is intended as a sharing of knowledge and information from the research and experience of Tiphanie Jamison VanDerLugt and her community. We encourage you to make your own health care decisions based upon your research and in partnership with a qualified health care professional.

* These statements have not been evaluated by the Food and Drug Administration. This product is not intended to diagnose, treat, cure or prevent any disease. If you are pregnant, nursing, taking medication, or have a medical condition, consult your physician before using this product.

The Book On Pregnancy AfterLoss

The Exact Life-Changing Tools, Techniques, and Supplements I Used to Go From Losing 5 Babies to SAFELY DELIVERING 3 HEALTHY BABIES ALL IN LESS THAN 3.5 YEARS WITH EASE AND CONFIDENCE!

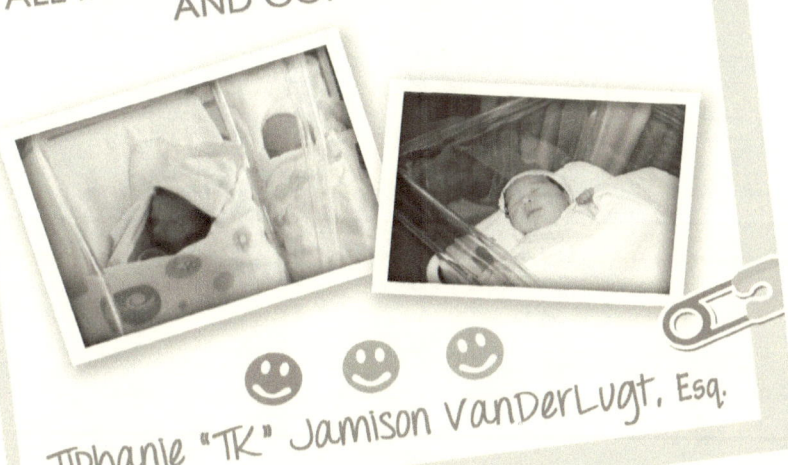

Tiphanie "TK" Jamison VanDerLugt, Esq.

Table of Contents

Introduction

I am not a doctor, nurse or medical professional. What I "BE", is a woman who knows the pain of infertility and the devastation and confusions of losing five (5) babies in a row. While I am beyond grateful, for the healthy babies I have now, there's not a day that I don't in some way, think of those babies that were needlessly lost.

Common Myth of Infertility

By far one of the most common myths of infertility is that if my body worked perfectly I would be able to easily and effortlessly become pregnant. The reality is that there are hundreds of thousands if not millions of women who have perfect bodies to ovulate regularly have no known disease or condition and still remain infertile it would file than that there has to be more at play than merely a healthy body. How is it that women with regular cycles, normal hormone levels, healthy eggs, and perfect sperm from their partners cannot get pregnant and stay pregnant and/or deliver healthy babies? What we need to understand and what I now understand is that the body is not separate from the mind. I submit the mind is 80% responsible for becoming pregnant staying pregnant and delivering a healthy baby. For some of you that may seem a bit far-fetched. I know personally when I think of women who work at work able to and effortlessly get pregnant and don't like children I think how's it possible that the mind be 80% responsible for getting pregnant staying pregnant and delivering healthy babies? Continue to read through this book and I will explain exactly how that is the case for the purposes of this paragraph, I will say that in order to get pregnant and stay pregnant and deliver a healthy baby there must be a significant and dramatic shift in your mindset. To become pregnant in the body you must first become pregnant in the mind.

All the tips in this book are the exact steps that I personally took to get pregnant and stay pregnant and deliver healthy babies as the title of the blessed title and subtitle states I lost five babies and deliver three healthy ones in a span of 3 1/2 years. You can see how remarkable of a turnaround that is. As you read through this book I invite you to open your mind open yourself it and challenging traditional ways of thinking. As a sad I am not a doctor and nurse or fertility specialists but what I am is a woman who was able to go from extreme loss to enjoying the love hugs and kisses of three perfect babies and a span of four years.

Think of your fertility challenges as a crack in the wall. You can certainly paint over the cracks, but at some point, unless, you go in and spackle the cracks, and address what is the cause of the cracks, merely painting will only prove to be a temporary solution. What you want is lasting change, and that is precisely what you will have with this book. Applying the analogy above… we are not simply going to paint, we are going to go to the root cause, spackle the holes, fortify the foundation, and build something MAGICAL! You can do it! I am proof that it is possible. If you need to, lean on my belief until you can muster up your own for now. By the end of this book, you will have easy tools, to help you become fertile in mind and body AND become a Radical Self Expert!

Many of the tips in this book may seem quite simplistic perhaps new age or even "far out". So much so that you may neglect to even apply many of the tips or quickly discount them. What cannot be disputed or dismissed is that I lost five babies and now have three; and I was able to do this in a span of 3 1/2 years. Never underestimate simplicity. In the words of Albert Einstein, quote "Make everything as simple as possible, but not simpler".

It is worth mentioning that while I include all of the supplements, practices, treatments, remedies and techniques that I used to quickly go from a "habitual miscarrier" and infertile to delivering three healthy babies, all were the result of my becoming a Radical Self-Expert. It was within this Radical Self Expert framework, that I was able to discover and uncover the next step, tool, technique, or supplement and take action. This framework/formula enabled me to create new ways of thinking and new point of attraction in my life. Once I was able to expand who I was I was able to expand what was possible. If you are approaching fertility with the idea that all you need to be is regular or have this last medical treatments or just use

IVF get greater sperm have healthier eggs I can say none of those things by themselves will result and healthy perfect babies. That is if you have been in this fertility game for longer than six months. Something happened that the six-month mark are you just be start to become jaded and doubtful and begin to really question yourself and that what each month passing those doubts and fears become a part of your mind that and really take hold of you.

I invite you to try it my way just once. Read through this book read and complete the action steps. Create a radical self-expert fertility mastermind. And go over these action steps with someone that you trust and who is also equally committed to transforming their lives and delivering healthy perfect babies.

Each technique and/or tool is divided into a separate chapter in this book. Remember you are a whole person, so mindset without action is useless, supplements without mindset is ineffective. They all work together. I was able to get the information because I was in action, I was able to withstand criticism and use the supplements, because I worked on my mindset. It is all connected.

I have attached everything that I did, said, and researched to this book. Some will resonate with you more than others which is absolutely okay. When you are a Radical Self Expert, you will know we can if something delete in fact part of being a routable self-expert is to know what is true for you. I offer these tips not to make clones of me but rather create a new way of thinking a new approach to a fertility journey. To at a minimum of acting and dialogue to show you what is possible. Some of you, may be thinking "well TK you were able to get pregnant I haven't even gotten that far!" I get it, believe me. However, even though I had five losses there were periods in between those losses in which we couldn't get pregnant at all- despite tracking our ovulation, taking our temperatures, and using a vision board. Not to mention the time after the loss of the twins in 2008, we attempted another round of IVF, which was unsuccessful and devastating; Our minds back in 2008, were still "hazy" after the traumatic loss of the twins, and the result was a big fat negative (BFN). The reality was we had a lot of work to do even though we were already on our self-development journey. I go into great detail on each of those mindset shifts that we have to make individually and as a couple.

If you would like some extra guidance and support it would be my absolute honor and pleasure to connect with you. I've created a free online action guide which includes all of the exercises and this book as well as exercises from the radical self-expert book and a complementary free audio to help you stay inspired and on track. Go to *www.TheRADICALSelfExpertMethod.com* to download these resources find more information and connect with me.

I am not a doctor, nurse or any medical professional. What I am, is a woman who knows both the pain of infertility and the devastation of losing 5 babies in a row. There isn't a day, that while grateful for my 3 living blessings that I don't think about my babies that were needlessly lost.

For those of us, that have experienced the pain and devastation of "infertility", somehow we are lead to think, that the cure to having the family we always wanted is to simply be able to ovulate, or take clomid[i], or perhaps a few rounds of the various assisted reproductive technologies. What my experience has demonstrated, is that for those of us with fertility challenges, the best and most effective approach to creating the family we so desperately desire is look at fertility as building a home. The blueprints are necessary, but on their own, not very useful; the supplies are great, but without a foundation, what will you build on? It is ALL connected. Analogously, for the fertility challenged, each fertility aid, technology, holistic approach, or otherwise, should be a brick in building the house or wall of fertility. Many of us, just long to be pregnant, we unfortunately, don't see past, the positive pregnancy test. Getting pregnant, staying pregnant and delivering a baby are very different things and each area must be addressed, just like the analogy of the house above.

What I have learned is that fertility is unlike any other condition, as it strikes at the very essence of who we are and what we were put on this earth to do- procreate. We are genetically designed to procreate and when that is threatened, what are we left with, who are we?

My mission in writing this book, is to share with you, my experience of not only overcoming infertility, but also transforming my life. I have removed all of the labels, descriptions, and their accompanying meanings, to create a life that I love. Applying just some and if necessary all of the tips in this book to create a new life, and healthy babies, will empower you to do the same. I am not infertile, a habitual miscarrier, patient, statistic, desperate, ungrateful, unexplained, unlovable powerless, and/or any other label that comes with being fertility challenged; and neither are you!

The last four plus years, have been the most painful, yet the most "lived" and alive I have ever been. It is because of those losses that I can now help countless others, not only with their fertility, but in life. As a direct result of the loss of those 5 angels, and the ensuing struggle to have babies, I am now a Radical Self Expert. I know me, trust me, and choose me.

Wherever you are in your fertility journey, you can do it! I am you, 4.5 years ago, searching for answers, full of confusion, jealousy, sadness and self-loathing. Through the use of the exact techniques, I was able to get pregnant, stay pregnant and deliver 3 healthy babies in a little more than 2 years. Believing that these techniques would work for others, I have shared them with a number of women through coaching. All of them were able to conceive and have given birth, and/or will give birth by the time this book is published. I tell you this, not to impress you or brag, it is not about me. As a person, who has "overcome", is it my divine duty to pay it forward. The inexplicable pain of a negative pregnancy test, or losing a baby, is something I would never wish for anyone to suffer. After the successful delivery of Bliss and Strycker, then Spring I vowed to make every tool in my fertility arsenal available to those, who were bold, brave and whacky enough to become Radical Self Experts and GET THEIR BABIES. You can DO IT! Open your mind, make the decision and act. I share with you, in great detail, exactly what we did, from the supplements and medications we took (prescribed and un-prescribed) to the most important mindset shifts.

Think of your fertility challenges as a crack in the wall. You can certainly paint over the cracks, but at some point, unless, you go in and spackle the cracks, and address what is the cause of the cracks, merely painting will only prove to be a temporary solution. What you want is lasting change, and that is precisely what you will have with this book. Applying the analogy above… we are not simply going to paint, we are going to go to the root cause, spackle the holes, fortify the foundation, and build something MAGICAL! You can do it! I am proof that it is possible. If you need to, lean on my belief until you can muster up your own for now. By the end of this book, you will have easy tools, to help you become fertile in mind and body AND be on your way to Radical Self Expert status! Remember, look at your fertility journey as a house. Build it with a strong foundation!

Once I healed my past, accessed my power, loved myself even a little bit, all of the keys to getting pregnant, staying pregnant, and birthing healthy babies were revealed to me. My babies are true miracles. All of the doctors said given my history of miscarriages it would not be possible for me to carry a baby to term. In fact, the cold hard statistics dropped with each loss. Many of the doctors, disagreed with my decision to take various researched supplements and alternative medicines, that historically been used to help women carry their babies to term and/or get pregnant. I refused to listen to the American doctors, who suggested that there was no need for prescription progesterone at all, let alone the dosages at which I was choosing to take them. Certainly, as many of you know, when you have someone of "authority", telling you no, particularly when you have a history of abuse, it is terrifying to disagree with them. However, I had an inner knowing and trust in myself, that for once in my life, I would be the "authority" on me. This is what I am offering you in this book. I am offering you, YOUR Power! You are more powerful, that you realize and my intention is that by the end of this book, you will take the steps to be a Radical Self Expert and have the life you so rightly and richly deserve!

As the subtitle suggests, much of the information that I found regarding herbal supplements, treatments and most importantly mindset shifts, were the result of my becoming a Radical Self Expert. Had I not become a Radical Self Expert, I would still be in a place of losing babies, languishing in desperation rather than triumph and celebration of Bliss, Strycker and Spring. I dive deeper into what it means to be a Radical Self Expert in a separate book by the same name, The RADICAL Self-Expert Method-The Fastest Simplest 7 Step Method to Discover How to Be Your True Self, Change Your Life Now and Be Happy Today!-The Easy Way! The harsh reality was that my life was simply not working, correspondingly, neither was my body. Whether you believe it to be true or not, our bodies' inability to function in complete health and in cooperation with our desires, is a reflection of the inner turmoil, upset, confusion, etc. Think about it, when you are in an amazing space, living authentically, no judgments, jealousies, stress at work, how do you feel physically? Do you not have more energy, feel lighter, your clothes fit a little better, you just "feel good", right? As noted by Dr. Bruce Lipton, *"The simple reality is that our perceptions and beliefs, whether right or wrong, are still going to control our biology. It is important for us to understand that if we change our perceptions, we can change our biology and our world."*[ii]

Many of you may be thinking, that you aren't going through a fertility challenge by choice, after all, who in her right mind would choose to be "infertile". I submit, you may not being necessarily consciously choosing to be fertility challenged. However, other choices that you have made in response to people, places and things throughout your life, are directly responsible for your being where you are in your fertility journey. We will dive into how some of the choices not directly related to your fertility, may be negatively affecting your fertility.

You and only you are the answer to unblocking every block to your fertility success. How exciting is that?? It is enough for now for you to know that EVERYTHING can change, because it begins and ends with YOU! YAY!

"I was exhilarated by the new realization that I could change the character of my life by changing my beliefs. I was instantly energized because I realized that there was a science-based path that would take me from my job as a perennial "victim" to my new position as " co-creator" of my destiny."

Dr. Bruce Lipton

As you have read and will note throughout this book, being a Radical Self Expert, was critical, no essential to my success in getting pregnant, staying pregnant and delivering healthy babies and creating a life that I love.

Being a "Radical", is a formula I created born out of my struggles with my traumatic past, unhappiness, emotional blocks, and need for practical information that I felt was lacking in traditional self-help books. I found myself coming away inspired after reading or studying a "self-help guru", but after a few days, found myself back where I started emotionally. It was like, ok, "I am ready, but how do I apply this stuff and what do I do with the fallout from those people in my life that are resistant to the new me?"

After the final loss of the twins in the summer of 2008, I was on a mission to create the life I wanted, so help me God. There were some bumps on the road, but my quest to get my new babies, was greater and more powerful. I studied countless "self-help gurus" and realized, that while the information they were offering was good, I had to be my own guru. From my journaling and notes, the Radical Self Expert Method was born. More than theories and positive thinking, this formula is about not telling you what to think or how to be. It is about you deciding what is true for you without the filter of your past, your environment, and/or thoughts, judgments, or beliefs handed down to you from your parents, caregivers, and experiences. The formula is to make you and expert in you! After all, who knows you better than you?

Each of the letters in Radical represents, an important key in the life changing formula. The formula can be used for anything from money, to babies, a new job, love, and/or happiness. It is ALL ABOUT YOU!

Fertile Mind...

"Within you right now is the power to do things you never dreamed possible. This power becomes available to you just as soon as you can change your beliefs."
Maxwell Maltz

Tip # 1 - Open the Mind to New Possibilities... New Ways to Doing, Thinking and Being

"Be open to new ways; sometimes newness just knocks on your door; welcome it."
Jonathan Lockwood Huie

We were trying all the conventional methods, and they simply weren't working. As Einstein, so eloquently stated, "Insanity: doing the same thing over and over again and expecting different results." Certainly Albert Einstein was a man of science, and I am sure was not faced with any fertility challenges, however, no one can argue his genius. Our ideas, prayers, techniques and tools weren't yielding the desired results, a baby. So the choices were either going completely, "fertility insane" or try something else. It was actually a relief to just say, "hey, this isn't working, let's do something different"; it was quite freeing in fact.

Prior to my losses, I have to admit I was not the most open minded person when it came to holistic remedies, alternative medicines, and new ways of thinking. However, I recalled an incident involving a client from my law practice. She always complained about EVERYTHING. I didn't want to be one of "those people" I despised. After all, she complained but refused to do anything about it. I would not let myself be one of the complaining-do-nothings.

Being open led me to so many awesome things, one thing building upon the other. For example, while researching alternative remedies and assisted reproductive technologies, I met, someone who introduced me to the law of attraction, Conversations with God, and other power of thought "gurus". That chance meeting between she and I, was the beginning of Bliss, Strycker and Spring. Had I not met her via a chat for women seeking IVF in Europe, I would not even begin to know how truly powerful I was and am, if I did not open my mind to the possibilities. At some point, you have to say, "What the hell? Nothing else is working".

It is because I opened the door to new ideas, ways of being and thinking, that I went from losing fives babies to now having 3 healthy ones, all within a 4 year period. Equally importantly, I found my life's purpose and mission, which is to share with others; how to be a Radical Self Expert, so they can have EVERYTHING they want and deserve, particularly those, who have a less than ideal past. I am proof that being open is not only the key to fertility success, but to life.

> *"Because I'm thinking in a broader way, I feel like*
> *I am able to make better decisions."*

Takafumi Horie

I invite you to do some serious internal unfiltered truth telling. Go ahead, no one can read your thoughts, and you never have to share with anyone what your internal unfiltered truth telling session reveals; ask yourself, is there an area of my life that I would like to change? Do I ever feel guilty for other people's feelings? Am I a people pleaser? Do I avoid speaking my truth to people, because I don't want to hurt their feelings? Am I kind to myself? Do I feel hopeless, worried, doubtful, angry, confused, or depressed? Are the relationships in my life healthy and fulfilling? Do I often feel like I am loving more than I am being loved in return? Can I say no without guilt, shame or judgments? Are there things that I haven't forgiven myself for? Do you wake up fearful that someone will see the real you and reject? All of these questions and so many more reveal so much about where you are as it relates to your fertility.

> **Action Step**: Ask yourself, if you are open to new ideas, processes, ways of being and thinking? Are you stuck in the idea that there is only one way to have a family and/or get pregnant? Ask your partner the same question.

"The key to success is to risk thinking unconventional thoughts. Convention is the enemy of progress. If you go down just one corridor of thought you never get to see what's in the rooms leading off it."

Trevor Baylis

Tip #2 - Decided to Do Whatever it Took to Get Pregnant, Stay Pregnant and Deliver a healthy baby + Took Action on that Decision.

"Remember, a real decision is measured by the fact that you've taken new action. If there's no action, you haven't truly decided."

Anthony Robbins

Many who are going through infertility think, by saying that you want to get pregnant, charting your ovulation cycle, and doing some internet research they have decided as a couple to do whatever it took to get pregnant and birth children. This would be about 30 percent correct. Desire, is certainly related to decision, however, what if, that meant, no sex for nine months, or moving to another state? Perhaps the decision would lead you to temporarily not having contact with specific family members, or saying no to people. Have you made that decision? As a couple, have you determined that you would take shots, live on one income, disconnect the cable to pay for a medication, or deplete your savings to have a baby? As Brian Tracy points out, "Your decision to be, have and do something out of ordinary entails facing difficulties that are out of the ordinary as well. Sometimes your greatest asset is simply your ability to stay with it longer than anyone else." I don't know many couples, who can say yes, to taking shots, or even possibly not having sex for 9 months, let alone, temporarily giving up an income, or depleting savings. You need to have that sort of commitment. It is not enough to want. There may be circumstances, situations and relationships in your life that may not be aligned with getting pregnant. For example, if you have relationships that are toxic, and unsupportive even though well meaning, you have to be committed to the decision to not be actively engage in that relationship, to maintain your positive, creative frame of mind.

Decision means, being an Expert in You and not rolling over and cowing to a Dr. who says it is not possible for you to have your child(ren). A decision only becomes a real decision with new consistent action. You may not necessarily have all the details in this moment, but you can still make the DECISION and be committed to it every single day. Action articulates the priorities.

"Using the power of decision gives you the capacity to get past any excuse to change any and every part of your life in an instant."

Anthony Robbins

DECISIONS:

As previously mentioned, after being introduced to the idea of the Law of Attraction, we "committed" to wanting children, but we hadn't reach that rock bottom point, and decided to do whatever it took to make it happen. I continued to practice law, though it was stressful and created immense negative feelings for me, with no clearly definable plan to leave my practice. Fearing being "the bad person", I continued to be in relationship with people, who were more than toxic for me. These are just two examples of how I hadn't decided to do whatever it took. I wasn't taking a new action to solidify, that I made a decision to "get my baby".

It is worth mentioning that we did try IVF applying some of the techniques I am going to share with you. However, even after becoming successfully pregnant with twins following IVF, we ultimately lost those babies because I had only painted over my cracks. I had yet to go to the root cause of my fertility challenge, fix it, spackle and then create something magical.

Certainly, every decision to do whatever it takes will look different. However, if you want to know whether or not you made "THE DECISION", simply look at whether you have taken a new action.

Decision #1 –Closed My Law Practice

Decision #2- Got rid of toxic people, places and things

Decision #3- Left the United States

What does a new action look like?? For us, it meant me closing my law practice, and having limited to no contact with those toxic relationships that were draining my energy. It meant, a move from the warmth of California, to the cold of Europe, to "breed"; a physical move mind you, in which, we had no place to live, no jobs and no prospects. All we had was our decision and the belief that this was necessary to create a cocoon of good "breeding energy"; Those are/ were huge new actions by any standards. Being in Europe less than a week or two, I was pregnant with our now healthy twins Bliss and Strycker. Do not under estimate, the power of a THE DECISION (new action) to have the family you desire. Once we made the DECISION to do what it took, we honestly looked around, and asked ourselves, "what in our immediate control, that is not in alignment with feeling good, or having positive energy? What doesn't feel "right" and who am I in relationship with that feels "wrong"?" Now obviously, something required some planning, for example, shipping the car, tying up loose ends, or even having conversations with those toxic people, before putting that relationship on an emotional hiatus during baby making time. However, with each decision, and the peace that came with it, we became more energized and more certain about the decision. Decisions by way of new action give life to the means by which to accomplish and succeed. Always remember, action goes before inspiration.

> *"The dreams I only thought about, the ones I took no action on,*
> *well they are still dreams. But the ones that I took action on,*
> *they are now a reality."*

Catherine Pulsifer

Action Step: Ask yourself if you have made the decision to do whatever it takes to have the family you desire? Look not at the fact that you "want" a family, or how deeply the desire runs. Your task is to look at whether you will do whatever it takes. What NEW actions can you take that are aligned with your deepest desire? Once you determine what new action you can take, TAKE IT NOW! It doesn't not matter if the action is small, so long as it is a new action. Do not worry about the next step. Take one action today, then another, then another. You can do it!

The conscious mind is the steering wheel of the mind. Comparatively, the subconscious mind determines attitudes, beliefs , how you perceive yourself and others, your values and motivations. The subconscious mind is developed via life experiences, beliefs handed down from our parents and environments, etc. Dr. Bruce Lipton, has termed the subconscious mind a tape player.[iii] There is no reasoning or understanding in the subconscious mind, it merely records information.

The subconscious mind is strictly a playback machine with preprogrammed behaviors that plays out frequently, when you hear someone say, "she really pushed my buttons!" Think of things this way, have you ever logically known something and did the opposite? Your actions were not guided by reason and/or logic, but rather, a feeling, a thought, something you were programmed to do because of your upbringing.

The subconscious mind occupies 95-99% of your mental real estate. Let us analyze the conscious/subconscious minds outside the context of fertility. If I owned 95% of the city, and you 5%, who would run the city? I would, simple enough to understand, right? It is the same for the subconscious mind and the conscious mind. Even if the conscious mind is operating at optimal speed and maximum capacity, it is still at best, only 5% of your mental real estate; this is why no amount of positive thinking without the enrollment of the subconscious mind will work. Essentially, you are trying to trick your energy, and since you are the energy, you know it a half-truth at best, and a bold faced lie at its most honest. How do you fix this, by getting your subconscious mind to cooperate with the conscious mind, i.e. clearing your limiting beliefs and programming, and creating new positive beliefs that support you.

Here is an illustration that led me to correctly understand how this subconscious/conscious mind thing works. After the last loss in December 2007, we decided to try IVF. While gathering data, we found a forum for American women that were going to Europe for IVF treatment. I me a young lady we will call her CL, there, and she mentioned in passing something known as the Secret. At the time, I didn't give it much attention, as I was focused more on prayer, and begging God to help me at that point.

After corresponding with CL for a few days, we begin to bond and she mentioned the Secret again and told me that she was able to use this "technique" to get 1200 bucks. Hell, I had to pay for IVF, so I was in! I went out, purchased the DVD and we watched it but fell asleep. The next morning over tea and coffee for Dutch we watched again and I took copious notes. I remember thinking, well that just makes sense, at least how the explained it in the movie.

We went out to my favorite store, The Wal-Mart Supercenter and got stuff for our vision board and immediately starting putting things on it. One thing we needed was a permit for Dutch to travel, because he was not American and didn't have a green card, so we put a permit to travel on there, & LOADS of baby stuff. We put 3 baby onesies to represent our triplets, the whole nine. We continued to dutifully go to church, visualize, meditate, and do everything the Secret said to do.

Thankfully, we received Dutch's permit to travel, which is a whole other law of attraction miracle in record time and were able to travel to Europe to meet up with CR and her husband; we arranged our trips to overlap so we could hang and support each other.

After 12 days or so we returned home, with a successful IVF trip to do the whole 2ww thing. UGH! Just as the Secret said we "believed", meditated, and visualized all over the place.

However, deep down, I had this ominous feeling. At the time, I was still practicing law, dealing with uncooperative clients, my ex was around driving me crazy and of course, those pesky ever present toxic family members. I wanted to be a "good" person, so I wouldn't tell them no, I wouldn't stand up for myself. What I would later understand, was they were being drawn to how I felt about myself. You see, I still had not dealt with the deadly 14. I felt less than half a woman for even using IVF, I felt guilty because everyone was against me, I felt unworthy because my family members were still using and abusing me. Self-value? What the heck was that, I had NONE! While my mouth was saying everything will be fine, my body, soul, spirit was like a troll in my ear- You know you don't deserve healthy babies, who do you think you are, you are nothing, everyone will have babies but not you; and this was some of the milder self-attacks.

Add to this, the seed that was planted by a "friend" in the forum about how all these other women used IVF and still miscarried and she herself had 6 miscarriages and on and on and I was ripe for a vibrated breakdown (more on the story of this "friend" in another tip.)

Suffice it to say, that as little things would come up, and I would try to gloss over there with my new "Secret" techniques, those think positive affirmations were INEFFECTIVE! In fact, it made things worse, as I got more anger for not being able to even think positive on a regular basis. Talk about monkey brain, ugh! When I would spot a tiny discharge because I was already coming from a place of unworthiness, guilt, shame, etc., it was blood and the end was near and I was surely going to lose those babies. As I reflect back, I no more believed that I would deliver healthy babies than I did that Charlie Sheen would become a priest. I was trying to "trick" myself into believing it was possible, but deep down, I was overwhelmed with doubt and anxiety. As an indication of how unconvinced I was that it was possible on a subconscious level, I predicted the day the babies would be lost in my mind. Wouldn't you know it, to the day, I lost those babies. The one day that was reserved just for celebrating me, the one day, that one of my favorite people went out of her way to show me love, I love those babies.

After my baby shower earlier that afternoon we were home and I was cramping like crazy. I noticed blood earlier, but tried to tell myself, it would be ok; there's the positive thinking again, I knew I didn't believe it though. Initially we went to the ER, the doctor took a test, and determined that the fluid was amniotic fluid, and an ultrasound revealed that my little boy's amniotic sac had ruptured and since his was ruptured his sister would have to be delivered as well, though she was completely healthy.

I left the ER, went home and showered and pretended like nothing happened- that was until active labor kicked in. Dutch and I got in my truck and we rushed to the hospital which was about 40 miles from my house. I tried not to push but did, and one of the babies was delivered in my truck, and was inside of my jeans. Finally we arrived at the hospitable labor and delivery and Dutch yelled for the nurses to help, and as they pulled off my pants, there was one of the babies. I was numb, and resolute. In my heart, I knew that I couldn't do get pregnant, stay pregnant and deliver healthy babies, despite my vision board, meditations and all the positive affirmations. After delivering the second baby, I was sedated, they took pictures and then took them away for testing.

Later test revealed that those babies were perfect in every way, and their loss was due to an infection contracted a few weeks earlier. More on that later in the book.

I share this with you not to gross you out or frighten you, but to share the power of the subconscious mind. You cannot fool yourself. Positive affirmation and the idea that the Universe says, "Your wish is my command", is not how the law of attraction works, particularly where you have a deep seated negative believe playing in the background of your mind.

It will always be easy to attract things like a parking spot, or a cup of coffee, because you have no negative thoughts about it either way. When it is something you really want, you have to get your subconscious mind on board, or you will be chasing your desire for a lifetime. This is typically the "inconsistencies" that people have with the law of attraction. For some things they can attract like snapping a finger, for others, it simply doesn't happen. If you can imagine, when your subconscious and conscious minds are not working together, it is like one foot on the break and one on the gas. You go NOWHERE!

Before I was able to even conceive of conceiving and delivering successfully, I had to get the subconscious mind on board. The Law of Attraction works every time. All you have to do is look at your life for evidence. It is totally impartial and makes no distinction between wants and don't wants. The law merely responds to your energy. If your energy is one of longing, desperation, disbelief and the like, you will attract precisely that.

"Positive thoughts have a profound effect on behavior and genes but only when they are in harmony with subconscious programming. And negative thoughts have an equally powerful effect. When we recognize how these positive and negative beliefs control our biology, we can use this knowledge to create lives filled with health and happiness.

Dr. Bruce Lipton

The wonderful news for you and for me, is that we can program our subconscious mind to work with us. By applying all of the mindset techniques I have shared with you in this book and my other book The RADICAL Self-Expert, you can stop the negative thoughts, release the old beliefs and patterns, and replace them with habits that will attract to you the life of your dreams. I've read that although humans have over 50,000-70,000 thoughts per day, 90% of those are the same thoughts from the day before. There is a virtual "Groundhog's Day" going on in the mind- meaning, we feed the same inaccurate un- productive, self sabotaging information over and over again. Those thoughts, become imprinted, more accurately cemented in our sub- conscious and then we wonder why things are not changing? I in- vite you to consider, how much you would accomplish and be, if you imprinted some productive, self affirming, personally empowering information? What would be possible, if rather than jumping to con- clusions, and limitations, you dwell in possibility and opportunity?

One thing that self-made millionaires, thought leaders, visionar- ies and average people living the life of their dreams have in com- mon, is the subconscious belief that they can accomplish any and everything they desire. From Dale Carnegie, and Albert Einstein, to Oprah Winfrey and Donald Trump, they all speak of having the mindset of possibility. As Albert Einstein has said, *"No problem can be solved from the same level of consciousness that created it."* Albert Einstein

HUGE ACTION STEP: What beliefs do you have around your life and your fertility? Take a sheet of paper and on one side, write a positive affirmation, for example, I am fertile. On the other side, right the thought that immediately comes to mind when you say that statement out loud. My subconscious thought was, "because you terminated a pregnancy when you were raped in your teens, you don't deserve to be pregnant". Yours may not be as harsh, but it is there.

Give it a try, what do you have to lose? Your way hasn't been working or else, you would be pregnant, so try it another way.

Tip #3 - I Didn't Focus on the "how" & Focused Only on the End Result-

"Once the "what" is decided, the "how" always follows. We must not make the "how" an excuse for not facing and accepting the "what."

Pearl S. Buck

"DO NOT EVER MESS WITH THE "CURSED HOW'S"

Mike Dooley

As human beings, when we want something, we try and figure out a way to get it. However, in so doing, we become so attached to our way of how it should work out, that we foreclose any other possibilities. I had to learn that the how in most instances is irrelevant and are generally based in a negative belief; typically fear and ingratitude.

Here are several illustrations of this point:

After the first 3 losses, we decided to try In Vitro Fertilization. Ultimately, due to cost and reputation, we selected a clinic in the Czech Republic. We had in mind that we would have triplets. Somewhere 3 was just our number. Following IVF we put back 3 embryos. When we returned from Europe and went to the local ob-gyn, he only saw one embryo. We were devastated. Our mood shifted from positive and creative, "oh gosh, what did we do wrong, we put 3 babies on the vision board, we manifested, we aren't powerful manifestors after all, here we go again, and so and so." Rather, than be grateful, we were down in the dumps. We went home pulled ourselves back together, and I decided that the Dr. (who was not friendly) was wrong. A few weeks later, we returned for another ultrasound and there was another baby and both hearts were beating. While we were "relieved" we were still not totally satisfied because we decided we wanted to have triplets; We believed (erroneously) that the <u>only way</u> for us to get pregnant and stay pregnant was with IVF. Note, that we foreclosed every other possibly of 3 babies by believing, based on our history of miscarriages, that we couldn't possibly get pregnant any other way. When we weren't able to create the *how*, which we thought was the end result, we were disappointed in ourselves, and in a very negative place emotionally. In our minds, if we couldn't create triplets, we were failures, so how are we going to be able to make it to term? All of those "crazy" negative thoughts, were based in fear, worry, doubt, etc. Sadly couple that disappointment with other negative emotions, we lost those twins. We were so fixated on having triplets; add that to other related negative emotions, and you have a prescription for disaster. You cannot create wonderful things, when you feel less than wonderful. What I learned was that you have to not look at how, but what! Follow what is your unique truth. I go into the detector of truth in the **RADICAL SELF-Expert Method**, but for the purpose of this book- remember what is true for you will make you feel lighter and expansive. What is a lie for you will feel heavy and contracted.

Comparatively, my pregnancy with Bliss and Strycker was successful, because I was in a different space mentally and emotionally. I had tools which I am sharing with you to manage would could be prove to be destructive to my pregnancy, if left unchecked. For example, at one point I started to bleed heavily during the second trimester. Now, I could have gotten down and say, why is this happening, I want a no risk pregnancy—a no risk pregnancy being the "how". Rather, than do that, I focused only on those babies being in my arms. My pregnancies were not the "perfect" uncomplicated pregnancies, that we saw on TV, or witnessed with our "fertile myrtle friends". Particularly, with a history of recurrent miscarriages, the threat to the well-being of the babies, was always lingering in the background; one cramp too many or too hard, a slight discharge, not feeling movement in an hour, if left unchecked could send me down the path of destructive thoughts, of which only loss was waiting. For this reason, you have to, no matter what lies in front of you, focus on the end result.

I don't believe that it was a coincidence that around the time, in the pregnancy with Bliss and Strycker, that I lost the other twins, that I began bleeding. It is particularly noteworthy, that the day this bleeding occurred, I was in a heated communication with one of those toxic people from my family. Up until that point, my pregnancy was relatively, uneventful time, minus the incredible nausea. When I started to bleed, my first instinct was to panic. My negative thoughts, ended there however. We went to the hospital, they did an ultrasound, and the babies were fine. They could not explain why I was bleeding, but I knew why I was bleeding, my thoughts were not where they needed to be, and I had understandable fears, as that was the time, when I lost the twins before; almost to the day a year earlier.

In that moment, I could have grieved, mourn, and disempowered myself and repeated another loss. Instead, I did not focus on what was happening around me or how. I focused only on the end result. Together, we talked about healthy babies and imagined ourselves playing with them holding them. We spoke to them directly about how excited we were to meet them. I continued to take my supplements to stop any cramping and just continued with the pregnancy knowing that all was well. That moment affirmed for me, that if I was not emotionally strong enough to even have minimal communication with toxic people. Correspondingly, I temporarily cut off all communication. I explained to them why and that at a later time, we could if, we both decided have a conversation about the breakdown in our relationship. However, I was not going to have that conversation until those babies were in my arms, healthy, safe and sound.

Here is the trick about the end result. It can be challenging as heck. Every time I went to the bathroom for a week, I was faced with my fear of losing Bliss and Strycker. Here are two things I specifically did, that helped tremendously:

(a) I asked myself, if I bled the entire pregnancy but at the end I would have Bliss and Strycker healthy and wonderful, would the bleeding matter? The answer was obviously, a HELL NO!

(b) I recognized that waiting for the blood to be gone, would only give energy and focus to the blood being there- not the end result of healthy babies. So I no longer acknowledged that there was bleeding. I referred to it as discharge and instructed Dutch to NOT as any questions about bleeding, spotting or anything else. I shifted my focus back to healthy babies, i.e. the end result.

As things come up in your journey to create a family, you cannot get bogged down in the mire of details, how's, what ifs, and why me. It will cloud your decision making, negatively affect your energy and the big actions you may have to take. If you are preparing for IVF, and you have only 2 viable embryos, focus not the fact that you only have 2 embryos, focus on the end result, a healthy baby. You only need one to create a baby anyway. If your cycle is irregular, and it doesn't seem like it will ever be, why focus on that? Who cares, if your cycle is irregular 10 times, because irregular cycles can result in very regular pregnancies. You have to know, that it's possible, when you focus not on how, and see ONLY the end result. How did I manage the "how's", I simply asked myself, if I bled the entire pregnancy, but would get healthy babies in the end, does it really matter if I am bleeding? The answer was HELL NO! Accordingly, I stopped focusing on the hows and here they are.

Now, going back to the first example of the desire for three babies; Remember, how I said, we were set on having triplets? We wanted triplets, because we thought, that IVF was the only way to get pregnant and stay pregnant, based solely on our history. We were totally focused on the how. When you focus not on the how, but actually on the experience you are seeking, you will get what you desired, in the easiest most efficient way possible. Within six (6) months of delivering Bliss and Strycker, I was pregnant with Spring, WITHOUT IVF, or other assisted reproductive technologies. So you see, we ended up having 3 babies after all. We were no longer focused on how. Heck, we were no longer focused on having babies at all when we had Spring. In fact, having Spring after the twins was an easier, healthier way. I was desperately ill with all of my pregnancies. So ill in fact, at one point, I was prescribed a cancer medication for the nausea. Further, with my "history" of miscarriage, putting that much strain on my body would simply not be wise. Ultimately, we received what we wanted, just in a different way; we now how 3 healthy perfect babies.

Stay away from the "how" you will have your family. You may think it will come via IVF, but don't see that as the only option. Some of you may think, if you could just get your cycle straightened out, all will be well. There are men, who think, "it's impossible because my sperm count is low". Listen, if you can have a baby despite any of those things, would you be focused on the low sperm count, a regular cycle or "old eggs"? What you want, is your baby, so the how isn't relevant. If you got pregnant with your last egg, sperm, IVF or donor eggs, would it matter? I promise you, it would NOT. Let go of the HOW'S. Holding onto how doesn't serve you. It only limits your ability to create and see possibilities. Remember, earlier, I talked about being open and new ways of thinking. Leave the cursed how's alone!

Focus only on the end result, because ultimately, all that matters is the end result. Now, this can be tricky, because our minds, will confuse the "how" with the end result. The good news is, we control our minds. You know the difference, and can take action based upon knowing the difference, that supports you.

I want to illustrate this tip in a situation outside of the fertility journey. Sometimes, it's easier to understand a concept when it isn't so close to home. Let's say you want one million dollars, so you say to yourself, I need to find a job that will pay me one million dollars. You try and try, and you can't find that job, so you give up hope. At the same time, you have an idea, for a new phone app. You have been giving away this phone app for free, but the idea with a little tweaking is potentially a multi-million dollar idea. You never pursue the phone app, because you are stuck on getting the million dollar job. A friend approaches you and says, someone asked them about your app and if it was for sale. You quickly dismiss your friend as silly and focus more energy and attention on landing that million dollar job. Later, you come to find out, that the friend's friend, was a developer with Apple. Do you see, that focusing on the "hows" will limit the possibilities? There are a million ways that one million dollars can come to you. You only saw one possibility and held steadfast to that. The "cursed how's", are dream killers, energy sappers and do not serve you in any situation, particularly pregnancy.

Remember, don't focus on the how it will come to be and see the end result. Applying this example again to your fertility, most all things can be worked around. If you don't have eggs at all, you can use donor eggs. I personally worked with a woman, 47 year old woman who had been through menopause and was no longer producing eggs. After applying the principles I am sharing with you, she was able to procure a donor who was her exact height, build, and actually favored her in looks; at minimal cost. Using those eggs, with her husband's sperm, they were able to have a set of twins, which she successfully carried to term and delivered. Throughout her journey, I worked with her on not seeing the hows and focusing on the end result. She couldn't be happier with her family.

> **Action Step**: Ask yourself if you are focusing on the how of getting your family? Are you being open to all possibilities? Vow to yourself and each other, that you will focus not on the how, but on the experience you will have in the end.

Tip#4 - Became Mindful of the 14 Mental Fertility Killers [Thoughts, beliefs, behaviors] and Developed Strategies for Managing Them.

Generally, there are 14 Mental Fertility Killers. Some of the Deadly 14 may resonate with you more than others. In my case, my history of abuse and neglect, indirectly, but prominently figured into my fertility challenges. For example, my feelings of unworthiness and being undeserving were formed in my early years as a direct result of the abuse and neglect. Those feelings were never dealt with and could be found in my relationships with others and myself. If you see babies as a blessing, and you feel at your core, that you don't deserve blessings, how can you possibly have the blessing of babies? Now, many of you think say, well, there are crack whores that "breed" like cats, and they don't deserve it. I say to that, (1) if they do have feelings of unworthiness, it may not show up as "infertility", it shows up in their ability to stay clean, form lasting bonds, be productive; (2) the more value or desire you place on something, the more you have to raise your energy, mindset, actions to get it; and (3) what does the crack whore's ability to conceive have to do with you anyway?

Now, on to the list:

1. Negative Thinking is a Virus
2. Fear
3. Anger
4. Unworthiness
5. Guilt
6. Shame
7. Everyone is more _____ than me; Comparisons and its ugly offspring Jealousy & Envy
8. Polarization... it's All or Nothing
9. Labels and Judgments
10. Your Feelings are Real
11. Associations
12. Fairy Tales
13. Shoulds
14. Like Everyone Else

14 Mental Fertility Killers

1. Negative Thinking is a Virus

> *"If you realized how powerful your thoughts are,*
> *you would never think a negative thought."*

Peace Pilgrim

How do you react to events that don't work out the way you planned? Negatively?

Make a choice to change your negative thoughts, before they spread like a virus into something positive. You have to stop the virus of negativity from spreading. If that means cutting off the source of the virus completely, DO IT!

During my successful pregnancy with Bliss and Strycker, I partially ruptured one of the placentas after vomiting. The blood was extensive and there was some clotting; which for many of you reading, know, clotting is never a good sign.

We went to the hospital, but the midwife (in Europe, mostly midwives delivery babies and do the first exam in labor and delivery), after the exam, said my cervix was closed, and both mine and the babies' heart rates were fine. She then dropped a bombshell on me. She told me, that because I was only 22 weeks pregnant, they would not take extraordinary measures to save my babies, i.e. stop any false labor, even if something was wrong. After wanting to punch her in the face, I looked her in the eyes, and told her, my babies were fine, and I was going home. She said she didn't recommend that, and attempted to sway Dutch, in Dutch (the language) to make me stay. I told him, "LETS GO!" I knew that staying in that hospital, when they said there was nothing that they could do, would only allow the negative thoughts, to take hold and spread. We recognized that being home, allowed me to meditate, connect with my Allies, be comfortable and manage my mood. I told her as I was leaving, "I will see you when it is time to deliver my babies." Now, I am sure, she thought I was a bitch and a crazy American, but I didn't care. I knew that negativity was/is a virus, and you CAN NOT allow it to spread, mutate, or anything else. CUT IT OFF at the source. I did. As you can see, my babies are fine and I delivered them by induction at 37 weeks.

It's important to be mindful of those negative people, places and things in your life. One negative thought is a seed, which spreads faster the blood through your veins. It is absolutely a VIRUS. Stop it in its tracks. As those negative thoughts come, switch your focus, back to the end result and ask empowering questions. For example, when we had the bleed, we said, "well, at least we get to see the babies again on the ultrasound" and "I love hearing those hearts beat". Yes, even though, we stuck to our mental guns and shot down those negative thoughts. You can too! You must, you will!

2. Fear

"Fear is static that prevents me from hearing myself."

Samuel Butler

Now, I am of the belief that fear doesn't actually exist; More on that proposition below. However, one of the largest obstacles for the fertility challenged is fear. I know that my fears ran the gamut. Challenges with our fertility, again, strikes at our essence. It is not like being homeless, or losing a job. Somehow, when faced with those obstacles, we believe, we can find shelter, we can find a job, but getting pregnant, staying pregnant, and delivering, or by some other means bringing forth life, seems next to IMPOSSIBLE.

Some common fears are:

- I am afraid, I will never get pregnant.
- I fear my eggs are old.
- I fear I missed my opportunity to get pregnant.
- I fear getting pregnant, because of my career, my job; what will happen to my relationship?
- I don't want to get fat; I fear getting sick during the pregnancy.
- I am afraid I will miscarry again.
- What if IVF doesn't work? What if it is hopeless?

What if, what if, I am afraid, fill in the blank.

The fear is completely paralyzing and sabotaging. I remember being afraid to "pee on the stick", because I thought I might be pregnant, but was "afraid" that I wasn't. UGH!

Interestingly, so many books and gurus tell us to NOT be afraid; but when you are bleeding heavily, and a dr. is telling you that, he will do nothing to save your babies, I think fear is a natural initial reaction; operative word being "initial". Two things developed from this: (1) Fear doesn't necessarily exist and (2) if you if you can't get with idea one, then there are tools to manage it. Except from my book: *The RADICAL Self-Expert.*

"So check this out... fear is oft en a misunderstood energy. Excitement and fear are the same feelings physiologically, right? Take this scenario.

Have you ever been in a serious situation where you should have been "afraid", but were totally calm? Most people talk about such an experience as being in slow motion, having super human strength, a sixth sense or guardian angel. In those serious and sometimes life-threatening situations, being "afraid" would be understandable, right? How can it be though, that if you were "afraid" you knew exactly what to do and remained calm, had a guardian angel or sixth sense? What if it wasn't actually fear but instead you were MORE AWARE? Let me explain...
Think about this, when a child gets ready to hop in the swimming pool for the first time, or on the first day of school, what does a parent say

to the child, "Don't be afraid". Consider this—maybe that child wasn't afraid, but just excited but couldn't in her/his young mind, "label" that feeling or emotion. So, when the parent says to him/her "don't be afraid", she goes, "oh, its fear I am feeling". Later, as she grows up, whenever there's a feeling, resembling that excitement, or an unknown situation or experience, she thinks, "I'm afraid". See??? She was entrained to have fear and be afraid when what she was experiencing excitement. Excitement is by its nature an expansive energy; it's a BIG emotion. Big emotions, are bigger, than what our minds can compartmentalize because they are expansive for a reason, right? They are to clue us to what is possible, to signal to us, that there's MORE than what we can see with our eyes or touch with our hands to light the fire in us, right?"

Excerpt from The RADICAL Self-Expert Method- The Fastest Simplest 7 Step Method to Discover How to Be Your True Self, Change Your Life Now and Be Happy Today~ The Easy Way! Tiphanie Jamison VanDerLugt, Esq.

Secondly, what I have found, is that there are tools that we can use to manage fear. Most certainly, the more you tell yourself, to NOT be afraid, the greater energy and more afraid you will become. The statement in itself is bringing about more fear. It is pointless to pretend that you're not afraid. What you can do however, is recognize that the fear is there and create tools to manage that fear.

In the five losses that we suffered the fear was a part of my every thought. To say that I was consumed with fear would be a gross understatement. Heck, I was afraid to even walk, with Bliss and Strycker after losing a set of twins preceding their pregnancy. Crazy enough, I was afraid to use the bathroom because I was afraid I would be blood and ultimately miscarry I was afraid to breathe too hard to move to heart I was afraid of everything. Unquestionably, these fears were totally irrational. The likelihood of my cervix magically opening up during the walk to the bathroom and my babies falling out is for lack of a better word RIDICULOUS!

This is the place that fear takes you when you allow it to rule your life. It takes you to insanity. Nothing creative and possible can come from a place of insanity. Whether you fear the judgments of others or you have fears surrounding getting pregnant staying pregnant delivering, whatever the fears may be they are self-sabotaging, counterproductive and utterly useless. I will not tell you that you will not be afraid. As a said I was afraid when I would see blood or if the babies did move regularly or even going to the hospital to make sure those hearts were beating. What I will offer you are simply some helpful tools began to manage that fear.

Before I share these techniques with you I want to the first briefly say that I believe that you emotion is simply energy plus motion. And what you have to do in some cases [particularly where the feeling or thought is extremely intense] is to allow yourself to feel that feeling to allow that energy to move through you to get it out of your body. With that in mind here are some techniques that I use to manage the fear.

Don't let fear catch you weak and unprepared. This is not to say, that you should walk around fearful. What you must understand, is that as you take action towards your desires, fear will come-up. Again, the trick is to take action anyway; I encourage you to come up with your own strategies but here are a couple of techniques that were very effective for me.

▶ Technique #1 I learned this technique from the show Lost. In this episode of Lost, Jack and his father were in the operating room. Jack was afraid to operate. His father then said, to him, it is ok to be afraid, but you cannot let it paralyze you. Christian, Jack's father on the show, then asked what it was Jack was afraid of. Jack told him then Christina told him, to close his eyes and feel the fear for 5 seconds or so. After the 5 or so seconds of really being inside the fear, Jack opened his eyes, and performed the surgery to perfection. This is an excellent illustration of emotion being energy + motion. What is truly awesome about this technique is that is not only lessens the fear immediately, in the long term, it will render the fear virtually powerless. It is a way for your mind and body to move that energy away from you. Now, after you have allowed yourself for ONLY 5 seconds to feel the fear, you must immediately replace it with something else. I used the affirmation, "healthy babies, healthy babies, healthy babies"; I would sing it and always said it 3 times. It is important that you pick something that resonates and feels good for you. It must be in the present tense and make you feel better saying. If it's sort of silly, all the better.

▶ Technique # 2 Fears, are 90% irrational; don't blindly accept them as fact. Challenge your fear. Ask yourself, what you are afraid of truly? If you are afraid that you are doomed to NEVER be parents. Challenging that fear, you know that is not true. There is no such thing as never. If you want to be parents, there is a way for you to be parents. Another fear may be, that you would have to use assisted reproductive measures to become pregnant. To this fear, I say, SO WHAT??? The trick here, is to not pretend the fear isn't there, but just to say to it, so what? Either way, barring death, nothing is going to happen to you that you cannot handle.

3. ANGER

"Anger is a killing thing: it kills the man who angers, for each rage leaves him less than he had been before - it takes something from him."

Louis L'Armour

"No man can think clearly when his fists are clenched."

George Jean Nathan

YIKES! This one is GINORMOUS! Is that a word? Anger is definitely in the top 3 in the hierarchy of mental fertility killers. So powerful is anger, that it creates a hatred on 3 levels- its powerful enough to cause of us to hate life, ourselves, and hate others, all at the same time. It is like the negative emotion trifecta. Anger is also very sneaky, it just creeps up without warning and the effects in most cases are lasting and/or irreparable. Being a California girl, I have always found anger akin to an emotional earthquake!

Many of us are angry over what someone said or did to us, or perhaps what someone didn't say or do. Initially someone's actions and/or inactions, created a hurt that caused us to feel sadness; which after calling a "friend" to vent about, pissed us the heck off and became anger, dare I say, rage!

Interestingly, unlike some of the other Deadly Emotions, anger is understandable; an insensitive doctor, an irritating unproductive co-worker, uncooperative insurance companies, do not bring up feelings of joy, that's for sure. We all have "triggers", so of us, a hair trigger, and some of us not so much, but we all have that thing that burns our butts! The key here, is how we deal with anger.

If you ever doubted the power of the mind's ability to affect the body and/or the connection between the two, you need only look to your response in anger. Note the physical manifestations of anger in a single moment in time, they are quite noticeable- elevated blood pressure, perspiration, flushed face, tighten jaw, headaches, "seeing red", we even refer to someone anger us, as "our blood boiling". If these physical manifestations are but a mere sampling of the power of anger, in a single moment of time, imagine, what a lifetime of anger can do to a person physically?

For the fertility challenged, anger generally falls into 3 categories: (1) coping with their anger by pretending they aren't angry aka DENIAL Denise; (2) pissed off Patty who is angry, doesn't care who knows it and is looking for every opportunity to unleash her wrath and (3) Rational Rita, who owns that she has feelings of disappointment, confusion, jealousy, and powerlessness, and those feelings themselves are the source of her anger. Anger, that is fueled mind you, every time you see a pregnant woman, here of a baby being dumped in the garbage, hear of a new baby's delivery at work; or worse, the insensitive comments of loved ones, family and "friends".

Here is my Top 10 List of Reasons the "Fertility Challenged" Are Angry:

1. Duh, we want a baby and don't have one!
2. Remember the crack whore?
3. All of the doctor's visits, where we have to share a waiting room with "those pregnant bit^&%# and the children she already has
4. The money that we are spending, that we would rather be spending on something like a vacation, new car, or anything other than fertility!

5. Shots, since when did intramuscular shots to the ass, become part of the procreation process? I don't remember that ever being in any lesson I learned in Sex 101: Where Babies Come From

6. It is just plain unfair! Why do I have to pretend to be happy for someone else? I am busy feeling sorry for myself... and NO I don't want to come to your baby shower, sheesh!

7. We want to move on, but the fertility journey demands that your life be "predictable".

8. Did I mention the crack whore with all the kids?

9. No one has answers?

10. Insurance? What insurance? This is all out of pocket in the great United States of America baby, at least before Obama became president.

I am certain, there are tons more, but certainly, these were mine! Feel free to add yours to the list. In fact, you will find, that it is very freeing and an excellent way to start to lift the emotional charge of that anger.

> **Action Step A**: Once you have completed your "anger list", then burn it and flush the ashes down the toilet, or throw them in a lake. Allow yourself to release it, as it is destroyed forever.

As previously stated, anger is reasonable, but your response is crucial to turning things around once and for all. If you notice 3 commonalities between Pissed Off Patty, Denial Denise and Rational Rita, was how removed they were from the effects of their anger. If Patty was aware of the impact her anger was having on her physically and in particular her fertility she would not be caring those emotions around with her.. Become aware of the effects of anger and how it is directly impacting your fertility and release it. .

In my fertility journey my anger was directed at myself. Admittedly I never considered the crack whore or a prostitute, or the chick on public assistance with 12 children. I was angry at myself because of my pathology. Blame and anger are often related. I blamed myself and was very angry for the things that I did in the past that I believed "caused" my fertility. I was also angry with God I'm sure on some level. I was offering up my best prayers. Dutch and I were going to Catholic churches praying to the blessed mother and we weren't even Catholic. Yet nothing materialized for us. I would have to say I most saw myself as rational Rita. Rational Rita, yes that was me. My quest for understanding feelings of "why me" confusion, and disappointments, were all at the fruit of my anger.

Understandably each loss was like gasoline on the California forest fire. Sadly my anger was totally internalized. Scientists have determined that one of the major impacts of anger on the body, is the release of hormones and chemicals, adrenal and non-adrenal. The adrenal hormones act on every organ, activating blood flow away from the vital organs and the uterus is not exempt.

By now, you are all familiar with enormous role, any semblance of hormonal imbalance plays. A woman's body under stress i.e. anger produces excessive amounts of adrenal, resulting in an adrenal deficiency, which in turn affects the thyroid; and wouldn't you know it, some common systems of a compromised thyroid, are short luteal phase, and no ovulation.

Emotionally, anger can lead to depression, or worse. Heck, some women have had to turn to psychiatrists and prescription medication to cope with the cycle of anger, frustration, sadness, depression wheel. Ironically, the medication that is helping someone to cope, may able be affecting her ability to procreate, which would in all likelihood end the situational depression in the first place. UGH! It was a vicious wheel of hell for me indeed. After one more BFN, and/or loss of a baby, I would pick myself up and attempt to move forward, only to find myself back in the wheel again the next month.

What I invite you to consider is how you can permanently get off the wheel. Maybe you aren't angry about where you are in your fertility right now. I ask you- are there other places in your life where you may be harboring anger? Are you angry with a friend or family member? Is there a co-worker that burns your butt? Does your boss drive you crazy? Is there a place, person or thing, that you immediately feel a physical manifestation of anger when confronted by it?

Remember I said, I have no expectation and neither should you that you won't ever be angry again in your life. Just become the master of your anger rather than it being in control of you.

Here are some tools to help you manage anger constructively and release it quickly:

1. Identify what your triggers are. What gets your blood boiling? Be clear on every trigger you can think of.
2. In the heat of upset, take a moment remove yourself from the upset and one deep breath, inhale for 3, hold for 5 then release for 4. Ask yourself, "What brought me to this situation"? What was I thinking at the time, what was I doing? How was I feeling? In order to know the cure, you have to understand the cause.
3. Talk yourself off the anger ledge. Remember feelings are not reality, they are just feelings. You may not know exactly what angered you in the moment. However, taking the deep breath will take some of the charge (energy and focus) away from the emotion.
4. The proverbial stop sign is always a keeper. When you are getting upset, see a Stop sign as a signal to stop the emotion from going any further. If you don't know why you are anger, chances are, it is your conditioned response to anger. We are trained that certain situations should enrage us and this conditioning is telling you to get angry. Using the stop signal will allow you to get some distance from the emotion. Ask yourself, now, am I angry or have I been programmed to be angry is this situation? Either way, the good news, is just by doing the analysis you have already taking the energy as least a little out of the anger.
5. Ask yourself a question, what else is possible for me? Just by asking the question, your mind will start to shift from anger, re-engage and try and find answer. Don't look for the answer, just ask the question and sort of remain in the space of the unanswered question.
6. Ask yourself, "who does this Anger belong to?" In my book, The RADICAL Self-Expert, I talk about how 97% of your thoughts, feelings and emotions are not actually yours. It may be that your anger, actually belongs to someone else.

7. Have clear communications with people. Be clear in what your expectations are, as often times, unclear expectations lead to disappointment, which in turn leads to anger.
8. Ask yourself, "What is really going on here?" What is happening right now, but state only the facts. No editorializing or "reading the other person's mind". Just describe what is actually happening.
9. Ask yourself, "What can I do in this moment to change my energy".
10. Run Your De-Way Clearings- This is a technique that I developed to release those yucky emotions. If you want more information on that, you can sign up for a free 7 part video presentation, **The RADICAL Self-Expert Method-The Fastest Simplest 7 Step Method to Discover How to Be Your True Self, Change Your Life Now and Be Happy Today!-The Easy Way!**

Again, I cannot say that you will never get angry again. What I am saying, is that in order for you to have your heart's desire, A BABY, you have to take control of your anger and feel less stress and upset; you must honor your body, by allowing it to be at peace and rest.

<u>Action Step B</u>: What are your triggers? What strategies can you have at the ready to manage anger before it reaches a boiling point?

4. Unworthiness

"Feeling unworthy is like putting a huge obstacle into the God force, into the life force which is everywhere. Self-worth comes from one thing -- thinking that you are worthy."

Dr. Wayne Dyer

Perhaps this is one of the most damaging of the deadly thoughts. It's so insidious because it is all encompassing of the deadly thoughts, guilt, shame, undeserving, and comparing. You have to see yourself as worthy and deserving of the family you desire. When you have feelings of unworthiness, you are forever seeking the approval of others to "make you feel worthy", and you can and will potentially sabotage your efforts, in life and fertility.

Here is how unworthiness showed up for me.

Eager and ready to "breed", I scoured the internet for something that sped up this baby making train. Not only did we order some fertility supplements for men and women at premium price, we both took home egg quality and sperm kits. Heck, we weren't spring chickens. According to the testimonials, I would likely be pregnant within 4 weeks of taking the supplements. With home kit results in hand, we were ready to procreate.

Almost immediately, I was in fact pregnant. I was both thrilled and slightly frightened; we had only known each other at this point for a grand total of 5 weeks. Shortly after learning of the pregnancy, the dr. that I had the checkup with contacted me and indicated that he would like to run more tests. The results were not necessarily conclusive, but given that we intended to get pregnant soon, it would be advisable. I told him, well, I was already pregnant. At which time, he told me, I had something called vaginosis (add footnote); an extremely common, not often recognized condition that was VERY treatable. He then prescribed a medication for me. Here is where it gets dicey. After learning of the condition, I did my usual net surfing and saw that the medication that is commonly used to treat the condition, is not necessarily safe for any pregnancy in the first trimester. Further, that while having vaginosis[iv] during pregnancy isn't ideal; certainly treating it in the second trimester is advisable to ensure that there are no teratogenic effects on the baby.

At the time, I was a HUGE prayer. Not in the productive, believing that God will answer me sort of way. Oh no, the bargaining, God is going to punish, please have mercy on me sort of way. Yep, the complete opposite of love, compassion and forgiveness. When I was silent, a voice said, DON'T TAKE THE DRUG. Yet, I went to the store and picked it up anyway. I didn't take it immediately though; but the closer I got to my next appointment, it began wearing on me that I didn't take the medication as told by my dr. Against, my better judgment, intuition, Source, God, or even science, I took the medication, because I wanted the doctor to like me as a patient. I wanted him to say, "Man, that Tiphanie is such a good patient, she does whatever I tell her, no questions asked." That's right, I didn't even ask him directly about the research I had found. I simply obeyed in an effort to receive recognition for being a good patient.

Needless to say, after a week of the medication, the symptoms of the vaginosis subsided, but so did those of my pregnancy. The last day of the medication, I happened to be in the bathroom and noticed some spotting. I knew this was not a good sign. I went to church, had someone pray over me, begged God/Source once again to give us a baby. Later that evening, in excruciating pain, and increased bleeding and cramping I went to the ER. An ultrasound revealed that there was NOTHING in my womb; which was confirmed by the attending physician you examined me later. More troubling, was giving my medical history in front on my new husband, and having his eyes (in my opinion) look upon me with contempt. I would love to think that he wasn't listening, but his questions, later revealed, he WAS listening, and listening with the ears of a prosecuting attorney.

Refusing to stay overnight, we went home, empty. My thoughts were racing, the unspoken blame was thicker than an iceberg. Many after a loss blame God, but in true to my emotional pathology, I blamed myself and determined that God had deemed me UNWORTHY. In those next hours, I played over and over again, ever lie I had told, every unkind word, and every sin that was supposed to be forgiven in my head. All of the nastiest vilest words that I wouldn't use on my enemy, I reserved just for me. If only I was better, different, more, or just flat out, someone else, God would Bless me with a baby. I blamed myself for not only being clearly unworthy in the sight of God but also for taking the medication. Interestingly, not once did I blame the dr. who prescribed it. I blamed me for taking it. Not in the healthy, take responsibility, lessoned learned sort of way; more of the "you are not ™worthy, who disgusting human being" variety.

Unworthiness is contempt for who you are. If you don't like you, how can you create positive thoughts about you? How can you be in a creative space?

5. Guilt

Guilt is the source of sorrows, the avenging fiend that follows
us behind with whips and stings.

Nicholas Rowe

Guilt is indeed a thief of all things good in our lives, including but not limited to fertility. My burden of guilt was guiding every decision I was making in my life. Unique to abuse survivors I think, is the level with we hold ourselves responsible, and simply let other people "off the hook". Somehow, we can excuse the behaviors of others, and recognize their humanity, but rarely if ever able to see our own.

My best friend says when you know better you do better. I didn't understand him at the time, but I certainly "get it" now. Growing up, I did a lot of "acting out", which was directly related to my abuse. I was hyper sexual, engage in risky behavior, was less than honest. Fortunately, despite my self-hating actions, I was still able to obtain 3 degrees by 27 and thankfully, most of those behaviors didn't carry on into adulthood. For those self-sabotaging behaviors that did carry over, I felt tremendous guilt. In truth, when I was "acting out", I was only trying to find love, and certainly no one was ever injured by my actions, but the guilt remained inside me, eating me alive. I would think to myself, " I shouldn't have been mean to this person or that person, or else I would be pregnant now. Why did I pretend to like this guy when I knew that I didn't?" I even blamed myself, for people hurting me during that time. If the sun didn't shine, it was all my fault. The more guilt I carried, that didn't even belong to me, the worse I felt about myself and the more difficult self-love became. When someone would ask me for something, I would just give it, despite it not being right for me, because I didn't want to feel more guilt; doing this cost me money, energy, friendships. I didn't know how, or even consider being honest for fear of hurting someone, thereby creating more guilt.

Worst yet, I felt guilt over terminating a pregnancy that was the direct result of rape when I was 12. Now, I look at my children or any other average 11 year old, and would know that delivering a child is simply not an option. However, as an adult, who was trying to conceive, I felt tremendous guilt over that. Many women have shared with me, that they too have terminated pregnancies for various reasons, and now struggle with that same guilt. Let me tell you, for whom that applies, let go of your guilt. Release it now. It does not serve you. You made the best choice you could with what you had at the time. Know, that your choice then, does not mean you cannot have children today. Perhaps you chose to give up your other child(ren) to adoption, or give custody to another family member; this does not preclude you from creating a life you want today.

The residue of that choice exists in your mind. Fortunately, you can control your mind. Your choice was not bad or good, it was simply a choice. The story around your choice, is what is keeping you in emotional and physical bondage.

You need to get, that your story about it being bad or good, is not serving you and that you are only powerful in YOUR life. Your story about the things you may or may not have done, is what is keeping you infertile, not a choice you made. By feeling guilty, you are judging yourself, as unworthy and underserving. If you do not deem yourself as a worthy person, then how can you bring forth something as worthwhile as a baby? Now, I realize some of you may go back to crack whore that has children easily, but again, what does that have to do with you? Secondly, she has her own "stuff" that she has to deal with. Thirdly, do you want to be that crack whore? Think about it, even though, she can have children, she can't stay clean to enjoy them anyway; isn't the point of you wanting to have baby(ies) is to enjoy parenting them, loving them, being with them? You certainly wouldn't be able to do that hitting the crack pipe, so let it go!

Many people hold onto guilt, because they simply know, no other way to be. Who would you be if you didn't feel guilty? Guilt is a way to NOT take responsibility for yourself, to not make choices that support you. It gives power to the "thing" and/or person you feel guilty about. You cannot bring forth life, carrying that around inside of you. It is taking up the space for self-love. You cannot love yourself, and not take responsibility for who you are today. Your guilt has condemned you to a life of infertility or the inability to ever create by any means available the opportunity to parent? Who made you the Judge of Baby Making? Your sentence to infertility hell, is one of your own creation.

"Guilt is the sum total of: All the negative feelings we have ever had about ourselves! Any form of self-hatred, self-rejection, feelings of worthlessness, sinfulness, inferiority, incompetence, failure, or emptiness. The feeling that there are things in us that are lacking or missing or incomplete."

Ken Wapnick

Action Step: Ask yourself, what you are feeling "guilty" about, not just from your past, but from today? For 24 hours, watch how you move about the day. Do you say things like, "It's my fault, I shouldn't have...?" Or do you do things, that you really don't want to do, because you would feel "badly" if you didn't do it? Just take note of how you are interacting with yourself and others. Do you find that you blame yourself for things, you really had no or limited connection to? Release it today, right now!

6. SHAME

"Shame is a sickness of the soul. It is the most poignant experience of the self by the self, whether felt in humiliation or cowardice, or in a sense of failure to cope successfully with a challenge. Shame is a wound felt from the inside, dividing us both from ourselves and from one another".

Gershan Kaufman

Often times, you will hear people use shame and guilt interchangeably. I can assure you they are quite different. As noted by Jonathan Bradshaw, "Guilt says I've *done* something wrong; shame says there *is* something wrong with me. Guilt says I've *made* a mistake; shame says I *am* a mistake. Guilt says what *did* was not good; shame says I *am* no good." Bradshaw(1988).

Shame is particularly damaging as it eats at your very essence of your being. In the end, if shame is allowed to take hold, you wind up feeling that who you are is just plain wrong. This is precisely what happened to me. I can't ever recall a time in my childhood and early adulthood when I didn't want to be someone else; a time when I wasn't ashamed of being me.

Until a few years ago, I was convinced that I was irreparably broken.

I don't want to get into the blame of and/or the origin of shame as the point of shame's creation is not productive or generative.

The challenge in dealing with shame is that no one wants to talk about it. It's hidden away in the secret place that those of us who suffer from that buried within us. Many of us, create an armor humor to protect us from being "outed"; or our façade revealed.

The awesome news is that, there is a way out of shame. The exit from the hell that is shame is to begin talking about it. YIKES! I know, it is the last thing any of us want to do. However, the "secret" is the shame. It is like an internal terrorist, sabotaging your future with perfectly timed attacks; the only way to disarm a terrorist, is to be proactive. In this case, proactivity means sharing your story. Share your story. You are no longer a victim of whatever circumstances that created that negative emotion. You have survived and now, you can choose to thrive and come alive. You can tell your story and heal others, rather than allowing you story to continuing telling you what to do.

My shame was so deeply engrained, that I knew of no other way to be. Until the point of losing my babies, I didn't even realize, the enormous price I was paying and the toll shame was taking on my life. Do I still wrestle with shame, absolutely, but I have tools now and I am sharing them with you.

With the loss of each baby, the shame grew. Rather than allowing myself to properly and lovingly grieve the losses, I was ashamed of my inability to stay pregnant. How cruel is that? My self-loathing and contempt reached epic proportions indeed.

Some of you may be thinking, how do I know if I have shame? Well, do you ever hide the truth of who you are, because of fear of being "found out and judged"? Do you ever get angry with your body because of its inabilities to respond to your personal demands of getting pregnant, staying pregnant and delivering a baby? What is your self-talk? When you have another BFN or a failed cycle of clomid, what do you say to yourself? I am by no means suggesting that you need to run out into the world, and put your life on display. What I am suggesting however, is that you be honest with yourself.

If you do have shame you don't owe anyone anything, but you do owe yourself awareness, so that you can make a choice that moves you towards the things that you want and away from those things you don't.

> **Action Step:** Get clear on whether you have shame from your past that's polluting your body. If you do, then make a choice to honor yourself and let it go. You are worthy, you are not bad, and you are deserving. Shame is not a part of who you are, but a result of programming. Release it, and make space in your body and spirit for your baby.

7. Me vs. Everyone…. Making Comparisons with Others and the Comparison Demons, Jealousy and Envy.

"If God had wanted me otherwise, He would have created me otherwise. "
Johann von Goethe

"Jealous people poison their own banquet and then eat it."
Washington Irving

Do you always compare yourself to others? If you do, it's high time you stop. I was the QUEEN of comparison and if I am not careful, I could very easily slide back to that throne. I compared myself to the people I cared about who were able to become easily pregnant un-intentionally, to pregnant characters on television, to people in chat rooms, strangers on the street. It was absurd. Oh, and of course, I compared myself to the crack whore with 12 kids. Who on their fertility journey doesn't?

Why are you putting yourself through so much of worthless competition? Frankly, it isn't even healthy competition. By making the comparison, you <u>magnify your perceived weaknesses and others' strengths and/or shrink others' weaknesses and lessen your strengths.</u> Do you see how, either way, you come out as "less than'? It is a mindset that you must shift.

> *"Don't compare yourself with anyone in this world...*
> *if you do so, you are insulting yourself."*

Bill Gates

Comparing yourself only drains your ability and power to create good things in you your life. Your success is limited to the success of those with whom you are making the comparison. For this reason, I caution against visiting infertility forums, and the like, which I discuss in greater detail in a later tip. Each and every time, you compare yourself, you give away your personal power, and the more you give of your personal power, the more insecure you become. Insecure people are not able to think for themselves, because their dominant focus is on getting the approval of others. When you are trying to create something as magical as life, you have to be able to rely on YOU. The feelings of not being good enough, unworthiness, inadequacy, and resentment of the success of will never get you to self-love, self like.

So, are you saying something like this?

▶ "There is no way, clomid will ever work for me, I tried it a few months ago, and it didn't work. Maria used clomid the first time and it worked for here, so if she used it once and it worked, then I know there must be something more going on with me.

▶ "There is no way, natural remedies can work for me, I am 37 years old, and my eggs are older. Besides, DH's sperm is on the low side. Natural remedies will only work Maria, because she is younger, younger women rarely have trouble and can get pregnant with natural remedies, 99% of the time.

Challenge these thoughts! Don't give in to them. Be aware as it comes up for you. Here is a trick that I learned to manage the comparison monkey.

1. Ask yourself, do you want to be that person? So when you compare yourself to the crack whore with 12 kids, do you want to be her?
2. Tell yourself, when you feel jealous or envy of someone's fertility success, say, "If they can do, I can too!" Look at it, as POSSIBLE!
3. Remember – 97% of your thoughts, feelings and emotions are not actually yours. So, as those thoughts come up, ask "who does this stuff belong to". If you want more information on managing thoughts, be sure to pick up a copy of my other book, *The RADICAL Self-Expert-The Fastest Simplest 7 Step Method to Discover Your True Self, Change Your Life Now and Be Happy Today!-The Easy Way!*

Jealousy is a blinding and powerful thing, particularly in the fertility journey. As I mentioned before, as I was going through all of my losses, two of my favorite people, successfully fell pregnant and delivered, and one was even pregnant for a second time with twins. It was on many levels quite painful for me. I would keep asking myself why them and not me? They already had everything, loving families, parents who wanted them, husbands' that were nice to them. Those feelings from growing up feeling like I was different, because I was "the only one" that bad things were happening to and whose parents neglected them, came up constantly.

Although jealousy and envy are generally used interchangeably they are quite different animals. Jealousy is more about losing what you have; involves feelings of betrayal, anger, uncertainty, loneliness low self-esteem and sadness. Envy on the other hand involves wanting with someone else has; more than wanting, but coveting what someone else has.

It is not uncommon to experience both as it relates to one's fertility. The fiends of irrational comparison wreaked havoc on me in my fertility journey. During my losses, one of my favorite people and Ally, we will call her Bentley was also pregnant. Her pregnancy, wasn't "planned", but I was so happy for her and her new husband; at least on the outside. On the inside, I was so jealous, I could hardly be around here. In fact, she delivered her oldest child, the day of my 2nd loss. OUCH! How could God be so cruel? During the dramatic loss of the twins, she was also pregnant. We later learned that she was pregnant with twins. Oh my gosh, I had to get off the phone when I heard that one. She understood, because she is wonderful that way.

My other, then Ally CR, was there with us, when we went to Europe for IVF. My jealousy, was eating me alive. She produced more eggs, so I was jealous, she recovered faster for the egg retrieval, I was jealous of that, she meditated better", visualized "better", seemed "happier". Gosh, just writing it makes me cringe. Unfortunately, it didn't end there, when we both came back from our IVF trip, she had a "better" doctor, her HPT came back faster, her beta results were higher, and on and on and one. Utter madness!

Throughout my losses and fertility journey, I would hate to go to the doctor's office, to have to sit there with the "pregnant bit%&es" in the waiting room. When I saw a couple walking, my heart would cry. If I heard of a child being abused or a baby being abandoned, it was sadden me. All I could think, was "why that "horrible woman" and not me"? I know jealousy and envy intimately! Can you relate?

What is true, it is absolutely normal. Don't beat yourself up, or feel like you are a bad person. You aren't. In my lifetime I have experienced both simultaneously. How many times have we watched someone holding their baby and wished it was us. The awesome news, is that there are tips to deal with the twin demons of comparison.

1. When you feel jealous, recognize what is underlying the feeling. For example, how does the other woman having a baby relate to you not having a baby? It doesn't, does it? Or if you are feeling lonely or isolated, recognize those feelings and connect with someone who can support you. Again, you can coach with me and/or lean on your allies. Where you may have feelings of loss, what have you lost? In my case, I lost 5 babies consecutively. However, my losses were not related to another woman having her baby? Her having a baby doesn't mean you won't have yours? Quite the opposite is true. If someone can overcome her fertility challenges, so can you!

Envy is much easier to manage, in my opinion.

> *"Envy can be a positive motivator. Let it inspire you to work harder for what you want."*
>
> **Robert Bringle**

2. Where appropriate and possible, become friendly with the person you are envying. I can't think of a single person who has walked the long road of the fertility challenged, that is unwilling to share what she did differently to be successful. Many of us are so eager to ensure that no one ever has to go through that again, that we are more than available to share our successes.

One thing that truly helped keep me on track was this notion. Positively framed, envy can be a source of great comfort that you are clear on what you desire. Envy clues you as to what is important in your life. I call it a not so gentle nudge of what is possible for you. You wouldn't have the desire, if there wasn't a way to experience that desire in reality. The wonderful news is that, "What, who and why you envy lets you know what you want in your life. It helps you realize what's important to you. You wouldn't feel this strongly about someone else having whatever it is you envy if it wasn't a priority for you. Here is the thing, if you weren't envious, then the thing you said you wanted, wouldn't.

8. Polarization… One or the Other! All or Nothing!

There's more than just black and white. Additionally, just because something may be black doesn't mean it's white. There are several colors in between, like blue, green, red, yellow, pink, brown, purple, and mauve, not to mention many shades of gray. Are you one of those who think "It's all or nothing", black or white? "I am either a success or a failure."

We know that there are certainly more colors than black or white. In fertility, too often, people think, that using supplements, or assisted reproductive technology is failure. For some of you, the mere thought, of using donor sperm or eggs, is unthinkable. I get it.

I invite you to consider broadening your possibilities. It's not true, that supplements or IVF makes you a failure. Or if you are a man, using donor sperm makes you a failure. The need for medical intervention means nothing. It is the story that you are attaching to it, that is the problem.

If your grandest desire it a family, it can't be, pregnant by March with no medical assistance or nothing at all. In fact, you may not need intervention or special supplements; we didn't when we conceived Spring. The idea is to be open, and not foreclose any possibility. You have to see everything, as a potential opportunity to create your family. For example, what if at the dr.'s office, you meet someone that went through your situation, and could share with you a cutting edge new medication that's available? It may be, that being at the doctor's office was the quickest way for you to stumble on some information, place, person or thing, that would help you get your baby- the fastest, easiest healthiest way possible. Just consider that. It is NOT this or that, baby without drugs or no baby; Natural vs. Unnatural. It's not one or the other. In life there are rarely successes and failures. Success and failure are not meant to be measured by the means by which you accomplish your heart's desire. "It's all or nothing" thought is only setting you up for failures. What do you call a woman who used assisted reproductive technologies, MOTHER! What do you call a woman who becomes pregnant naturally MOTHER! Keep that in mind! ☺

9. Labelling and Judgments

Judgment only creates separation between you and your desires.

How often do you use an adjective to describe yourself? More specifically, how often do you judge your behavior and attach a name to it.

- I am a loser, I am ugly, I am fat, I am infertile, I am stupid.

Judgments...

The funny thing is, we think that by judging something, it will create the change in our behavior, circumstance or situation. When has that ever worked long-term? Whatever we judge someone else or something, we cement that judgment in our lives and keep ourselves stuck.

Our judgments and labels are our unfortunate filters. We use them to make sense of things in the world. When you judge yourself as bad or infertile, hopeless, habitual miscarrier, broke, or needing to do something other than be who you are—how does that feel? Heavy, right? Do those judgments create possibilities? Or do they make you want to run and hide? Judgments are about fixed ideas and belief systems. Since, they are fixed, by nature; they prevent other possibilities from being and you experiencing those possibilities. Whether you are judging others, or yourself, when you engage in such behavior, you are solely focused on what you are not, rather than what you are. Judgments limit your choices; and choice is your trump card. Also, judgments are merely a summary of other people's feelings, ideas, and beliefs, which you have been conditioned to believe are your own. They are not yours and in no one serve you. How does this affect your fertility? Well quite simply, if you make choices, then label or judge them as bad, stupid, or ridiculous, (1) you are not able to see all the possibilities of creating your family, (2) you are deeming yourself unworthy and undeserving again, and (3) you won't take a specific action that would lead to you enjoying the life you desire because how can you trust yourself, if you have judged you as "stupid"? These are but a few reasons why judgments and labels are toxic.

More specifically, I hear women judge themselves because they are using assisted reproductive technologies to create their families. Sadly, IVF, IUI, and the like, remains looked upon as freakish and/or "unnatural". Many couples have judged it as shameful and as such will miss out on the opportunities of having the family they always dreamed of. This is also quite common among men, with a lower sperm count. These men have judged themselves as "less than" simply because they may require so additional assistance impregnating their partners and/or wives.

For those who have resistance to and/or judgments about ART, sperm donation and the like, ask yourself, are babies shameful? Do you ever look upon a newborn and think; you should be ashamed of how you have come to be? Of course not! Judgments merely keep you stuck and stand between you and the life of your dreams.

As Dr. Wayne Dyer so eloquently points out, *"Judgments prevent us from seeing the good that lies beyond appearances."* Does the use of any technology make that baby or babies less of a miracle? When you remove the label for judgment the use of IVF, I UI, clone my goal or any other medical assisted reproductive technologies becomes an opportunity to be parents, nothing more, nothing less.

So how do you remove the labels, thereby remove the negative story, just stop using them. When something happens, don't label it as good or bad, it just is. Don't judge other and don't judge

48

yourself. I can guarantee, you will feel lighter and see the world differently.

"It took me a long time not to judge myself through someone else's eyes."
Sally Field

> **Action Step**: Go 24 hours without labeling something as good or bad and note how you feel. Also, note how often other people label. It will be quite an eye opener indeed.

10. Your Feelings as Reality

Feelings are not facts. If you believe your feelings blindly and live as if they are real, you will suffer numerous setbacks. Feelings are only thoughts you have given meaning. They are NOT real.

Do you say things like, "I feel bad. Therefore, I must be bad" or, "I feel like a loser. Therefore, I must be a loser." Applying this to fertility challenges, "I feel bad, therefore I must be bad, and that's why I can't have children. Feeling powerless doesn't make you powerless and feeling hopeless doesn't make you hopeless. There is always a way, when you are open to the possibilities to having the family you desire. The fact is, you can create the family you want, if you decide, be open and take action. Those actions may be, acupuncture, a surrogate, IVF, or progesterone, but it is NOT hopeless. Seeing feelings as reality, merely, distort the situation, and create permanent obstacles to a solvable situation. Before you blindly go off believing you are bad, because you feel bad, challenge those feelings and question them. When you feel hopeless, ask yourself, "is there any means by which I can have a family?" There will always be one. Another question is, "What else is possible here?" Perhaps there's an option, not one you have entertained, or believe you could afford, but there is a way. Follow that with more questions. Don't try and solve the problem as you see it, just ask the question, "is there ANY way", when you think in questions, your mind searches for the answers. Challenge your feelings by questioning them!

11. 'Shoulds'

Some people surround themselves with 'Shoulds'.

- ▶ "I should have started trying to get pregnant before 40."
- ▶ "I should be pregnant by now."
- ▶ "I should be married by now."

Are you a "shoulder"?

'Shoulds' are the unreasonable and unjustifiable demands you place on yourself. A 'should' represents what you think you ought to be doing, rather than what you are doing.

How do you feel, when you know you 'should' be doing something but are not doing it? Perhaps, you feel inadequate, hopeless, frustrated, and/or guilty? Yes, the list can go on.

So, what are your plans to get rid of the 'shoulds'? It's easy. Just change the 'should' to 'will', or 'could'.

- ▶ "I could do this."
- ▶ "How could I do this?"
- ▶ "I will do that."

Or my personal favorite, "What else is possible for me?""

12. Fairy tales, Perfection....and They all Lived Happily Ever After?

Many of us, coast through life, believing, that when we are "ready" for a baby, our minds, bodies, and spirit, irrespective of how we have treated them, will respond. NOT! Wouldn't it be wonderful, if we could meet someone fall in love, have a baby on command, and live happily ever after? This idea, that there's a "perfect" time, or asking "why me", is keeping you from creating your family. If your focus is on the imperfection, you are in a place of being ungrateful, and limiting the possibilities.

"People throw away what they could have by insisting on perfection, which they cannot have, and looking for it where they will never find it."

Edith Schaeffer

Rather than seek perfection, enjoy the imperfections. Those imperfections are awesome lessons that were chosen for you. My pregnancies weren't perfect, I didn't receive exactly what was on my vision board, i.e., triplets 2 boys and 1 girl. When I just let go, I was able to get pregnant, stay pregnant and deliver 3 healthy babies, in the healthiest safest way for them and myself. I realize now, that had I known about this Fertility Mental Killer, I am sharing with you, I would have been able to enjoy those babies faster; I would have been able to get out of my own way. While those losses, were excruciatingly painful, it is from those moments, that I can now share my experiences with you. Let go of the ideas of the perfect life, with the perfect way of conceiving, the perfect pregnancy, and the perfect baby. Focus, on imperfectly having your family that you can love and enjoy perfectly as only you can.

13. Associations

It is important to be mindful of whom you share energy with. As Magic Johnson pointed out:

"If people around you aren't going anywhere, if their dreams are no bigger than hanging out on the corner, or if they're dragging you down, get rid of them. Negative people can sap your energy so fast, and they can take your dreams from you, too."

Magic Johnson

As you will find in the tips to follow, negative energy can sneak in through a variety of channels. Friends, family and loved ones, tend to be excellent hosts for negative energy, because oftentimes, the negativity is unknowing, ever so subtle, and wrapped in love and concern. Guard your energy, you are the only gatekeeper and your life depends on it. Remember, like attracts like, so remain in the expansive space of possibility. I am often asked, if negativity and sabotage are so subtle, how will you even know when it's here. Again, in my book **The RADICAL Self-Expert**, I go into greater detail about the internal detector of truth. For the sake of this book however, I will share with you this principle.

Lies: When you receive data from some person place or thing, if it is not true, you will feel a sense of heaviness, confinement, weighted. The energy is like a dense fog. If upon hearing something, you feel heavy, contracted, and dense, it is a lie for you.

Truth: Comparatively, when something IS TRUE for you, you will feel light as a feather, dare I say, fluffy, and expansive. It is important to note, the feeling associated with your truth is neither good nor bad necessarily, it's just heavy or light.

Notice the word enlightenment has come to represent an awakening to or illumination of, the truth. Note, that the word, has LIGHT in it. The word is not *enHEAVYment*, right?

You are the answer to every question you have. Check in with yourself. When you talk with a person, even though it is a close friend or family member, ask yourself, "how do I feel?" Do I feel light and expansive? Not good or bad, positive or negative, but just light and expansive. Now, compare it to whether you feel heavy and contracted. For example, when you talk with a friend about IVF or using a surrogate, and they hit you with a tidal wave of questions, check in with yourself. How do you feel when this person is saying these things? You don't need to overanalyze, just be aware of your immediate response to the questions. Do you feel light and open? Or do you feel like you want to crawl into your shell, or someone is squeezing you energetically.

The people, with whom you spend your time, impact your energy. Especially in your fertility journey, the importance of surrounding yourself with pleasant, authentically happy people is crucial. I refer to them as Allies in another tip and give a sort of Ally guide list as well. Your Allies are those people that help you see all of life's possibilities, make you smile, empower and encourage you. They do not rain on your parade with unsolicited advice and commentary on your decisions and choices.

Watch out for the moaners and whiners. We all know a few or in my case, 10 or 20. They are always putting people down, don't like others being successful, are jealous, "preparing for the worst but hoping for the best", negative thinkers. Phew! Just typing that brings my energy down a level. Such people are energy vampires, will suck the very life out of you, bleed you dry and take you a million miles off the path to success. They are recruiters for the "non-achievers, life is unfair, powerless, wait and see club". Don't believe the hype; don't drink the Kool-Aid. More importantly, don't hop in the pool with them, to rescue them from themselves. It is a waste of energy! You are responsible for your power and them for theirs.

"You must constantly ask yourself these questions: Who am I around? What are they doing to me? What have they got me reading? What have they got me saying? Where do they have me going? What do they have me thinking? And most important, what do they have me becoming? Then ask yourself the big question: Is that okay? Your life does not get better by chance, it gets better by change."

Jim Rohn

To ensure you are running with the right "association", here are some things to remember:

1. You have the power to choose who you hang out with. Ideally, you want happy, vibrant and expansive people. Think of your life as a corporation. Who do you want on your board of directors? You want people who bring joy, love, support and empowerment, not negativity, criticism and insecurity.

2. If you have good friends who are negative and yet you want to hang around them, ask yourself why? What are you holding onto? Get clear on whether it is possible to have this person or persons in your life, and keep your energy where it needs to be.

3. If you decide that you want to keep someone around, who is a "negative Nellie", at minimum express to her/him/them, how their negative is having an impact on you and your fertility success. Don't make them wrong, simply say, "My experience is _____. What I would like us to is _____. Can we agree that we will not _____ together? If she/she/ they authentically love you, they will respect and honour your honesty.

   If you get a negative reaction, then you have your answer right there, and move on Martha, move on! If you find, that the negativity is intermittent or related to certain topics, have a conversation about that. If it becomes too much, then you have to make the choice to support yourself. It is better to catch the wave back to shore alone, than find yourself in a tsunami of negativity.

4. Don't think for one second, that these "rules" aren't applicable to family members. Heck, in most cases, they are the biggest negativity offenders. Your more mature family members have beliefs, attitudes and behaviours that have been conditioned for years. Acknowledge where they are emotionally in their lives, and institute a negativity filter. When all else fails, limit contacts, or subject matters that are triggers for "stinking thinking".

5. Keep in mind – You are not bad, selfish, or evil, for choosing your own happiness and peace of mind. If you don't you have nothing to give to anyone else anyway. Love yourself enough to be in a loving positive association, rather than in the non-achievers club.

14. Like Everyone Else

"Be daring, be different, be impractical, be anything that will assert integrity of purpose and imaginative vision against the play-it-safers, the creatures of the commonplace, the slaves of the ordinary."

Cecil Beaton

Do you cringe at the thought of "standing out" or being different? For much of our lives, we just want to "fit in" and go to extensive lengths to do so. In school, people try and pick the "right" clothes, and hang with the "right" crowd. Being different is certainly not desirable at that age; in fact those that are different, are mercilessly ridiculed and ostracized. Given that it is a basic need to "belong", it is not surprising how strongly the desire to "be like" other people is; connection is not only understandable but in human DNA. Sadly, the desire to "fit in" doesn't end in school. Adults find themselves often ostracized for self-expression.

When it comes to creating the life of your dreams, and in this instance a family, being different is not only desirous, but necessary.

When you are simply going along to get along and belong, all critical thinking goes out the window. You stop asking questions. You unwittingly begin substituting the judgment of others for your truth. . As previously indicated, being a Radial Self Expert, means knowing what is true for you. If you are just trying to "fit in", you're not following your unique truth.

When I tried to not make waves, and just "fit in", the result was catastrophic, resulting in 5 lost babies. When I followed my own knowing, the result was Bliss, Strycker and Spring. , I chose to take medications, that weren't considered standard protocol for my "diagnosis" or lack thereof. My medical records did not reflect any auto-immune issues, which would warrant the administration of a steroid. However, I brought the information that I found from my research and told the doctors, and said, "I realize that this was not typically done, but I AM going to do it anyway, it can only help and can't hurt." Obviously, I was correct, as evidenced by Bliss, Strycker and Spring. I was willing to be different, to not fit in, and do it my way. The greatest and most powerful thing on earth you have, is YOU; your ability to know you, trust you and your body. You hold the key to unlocking your fertility and success. I am neither advocating nor suggesting that you go out and try untested, unproven therapies. **I am not a medical doctor and I don't play one on TV.** In fact, here is a great place for the disclaimer: The information here is provided for informational purposes only and is not a substitution for medical advice. To See the Disclaimer in its Entirety, Go to Endnotes[v]. Do your research and then ask yourself the question "is this true for me?" Don't worry about who did it before you, whether your friends, family members or those people in the "forum" are familiar with it. You choose to stand out, so that you can stand up for you and your baby. In your fertility journey, give yourself permission to be different. You don't have to try for a year naturally before moving to IVF, where you feel that IVF is right for you. If you decide you don't want to try IVF and would rather go the natural route, with perhaps alternative treatments, such as Reiki, or some other form of healing. DO IT! Be different! Don't follow conventional wisdom. Heck, I always think, if I am going down, I am going down by my own hand! Never again, will I place my fate in the hands of strangers, like I did with those 5 babies I lost.

Certainly, I am not advocating a reckless disregard for your health and/or safety. What I am saying is to listen to you and even if you don't know of anyone on the planet doing what you are doing, check in with yourself, and find your truth! No one knows what you know, NO ONE!

Tip #5 - Made A Point to Feel Expanded, Generative with Tons of Laughter and Smiling (watched funny movies and TV & completely turned off the news)

"Be vigilant; guard your mind against negative thoughts."

Buddha

While we think that we are not susceptible to our environments, we absolutely are! For that reason, we must be the gatekeepers of our minds, hearts and energy. Where attention goes, energy flows, and we certainly don't want negative energy flowing while we create a baby. Negativity is insidious, and it sneaks into our minds, without our awareness at times. It comes in the form of news, daily newspapers, various TV shows, "friends", and family members. While we cannot change what's on the news, what we can change is how we are interacting with it. For example, during my pregnancy with Bliss and Strycker, I didn't watch any news programs, didn't read the papers, and remained "blissfully ignorant"- pun intended. Further, I didn't watch shows about women you had complications with their pregnancies, sick children or babies, telethons, starvations, or anything else, that would bring feelings of sadness. If an episode of Grey's Anatomy, or some other show, had babies in it, I skipped that episode. I made sure to not allow those things to even plant the seed in my VERY susceptible subconscious. To this day, I don't watch the news, unless there is a positive story. Some of my favorite pregnancy shows were, Frasier, Two and a Half Men, Malcolm in the Middle- keep in mind, most of those shows were off the air, so I had to get the DVDs, or watch reruns; which was fine, because I laughed A LOT! Laughter is awesome for good energy. It is indeed an excellent prescription for negative energy. For those non-sitcom shows, I did watch, they were either unrelated to pregnancy and/or were science fiction, for example, Lost.

Action Step: Make a stand for yourself and your baby, and choose to not give ANY attention to negativity. It is not welcome in your presence. Where have you been allowing negativity into your presence? How can you respond differently? Take control, it is a choice. If someone is speaking about their pain and heartache, you can either choose to get in the negativity with them, offer a solution or remove yourself from the situation. YOU CAN CHOOSE!

Tip#6 - Stopped using the Labels- Infertile, Habitual Miscarrier, High Risk, Low Sperm etc.+ Only Discussed the "Label" When the Doctors Asked

"Every human being is the author of his own health or disease."

Buddha

"The words "I am" are potent words; be careful what you hitch them to. The thing you're claiming has a way of reaching back and claiming you."

A.L. Kitselman

Look at the word, Dis-ease, it is simply "Dis- ease", i.e., not being at ease. Remember, I said, emotion is merely energy in motion. Well, similarly sickness is a negative energy state. It is a vicious cycle that begins in our minds and when the belief is held strongly enough for a significant length of time, it manifests. By way of example, let's look at an average stomach ache. If you have a firm belief in illness and you feel a stomach churning coupled with a headache, your mind, immediately goes to "I am coming down with something." Perhaps, you hear at the office or from a loved one that the flu "is going around", so you tell yourself, "I must have caught something, I must have caught the flu". The result, you ultimately end up with the flu, as your "perceived" sickness has taken root. Fear and negative thoughts, of being ill and having the flu, reinforces your belief that you are in fact ill, which in turn brings more symptoms of the disease and/or illness. It is a negative loop that we get caught in.

Comparatively, what if you were coming from a personal belief of wellness? Instead of you immediately jumping to illness, you say, "This is a physical expression of some energy imbalance, i.e., you are feeling warn down from stress at work, or at home, you have been arguing with your significant other, or you haven't been practicing radical self-love. Since your belief was rooted in energy, you wouldn't immediately go to illness, rather it would go to seeing yourself vibrant and well.

Consider the following:

1. Your body is designed to heal itself.
2. Doctors & scientists are only equipped with knowledge gathered & based upon past perceptions and observations- still they are NOT all-knowing. There are instances every day, including myself, that cannot be explained in medical terms. I personally can attest to 3 miracles, right off the top of my head. Interestingly, because these instances defy medical reasoning, they are labeled miracles.
3. Miracles, are merely the acceptance and acknowledgement of the perfect health and well-being as your natural state.
4. Focusing only on your illness, pain, and/or "Dis-ease", will only bring more of the same. You have to get out of the cycle of illness mentally.
5. When you focus on miracles, that attention merely expands the possibilities of more miracles.
6. Perfect health from where you are, is possible, if that is truly your focus, desire and belief.

So you see, if you label yourself as PCOS, or Peri-menopausal, you will only attract more or those symptoms, further cementing that belief. Once that belief truly takes root, it is more challenging to dispense of. What you want to do, is throw away that label once and for all, and see yourself as perfectly fertile. Now, I get that for someone of you, perfectly fertile, may mean the use of IVF, or other reproductive technologies. Perfect fertility simply means, the ability to bring forth life. DO NOT focus on the how. Perhaps if you choose a surrogate, you still have to produce eggs, or if you use IVF, or IUI, you still have a role to play, in which your physical health is key. You are PERFECTLY fertile, where ever you are. The key here is, to focus on health, see yourself in absolute perfection and know that your body has the power to heal. When you feel an "expression" of a health challenge, i.e. a headache, cramps, etc. check in with yourself. Ask yourself, what is my body trying to tell me? Do I need more rest, less stress? Do I need to have a conversation with someone to clear the air? Do I need to not converse with this person again?

I remember, in all of my losses, whenever I had a communication with my ex-husband, I started to bleed. Now, many of you will say, that is unbelievable. Sadly, during those losses, I didn't understand, that my spirit, my mind, my emotional energy, was trying to speak to me. I was unable to listen because of all the baggage. I would be fine, then one conversation with him, and I would bleed. You see, the energy was negative, and brought up all of the yucky feelings from my childhood and from my past. Immediately, I would have those feelings of being undeserving and unworthy and my physical body would react. As a result of the fear and already existing doubts, more negative energy was like gasoline on a flame. By comparison, all of those "negative" energy people had little to any contact with me during my other pregnancies. In fact, they didn't even know I was pregnant until after I delivered! I was carrying precious cargo and I refused to allow them to stain it with their drama. As a Radical Self-Expert, I knew my limitations and weaknesses as it related to being sucked back in to that abyss of madness. I took the necessary steps to protect my babies.

Equally importantly, we never discussed the medical label with anyone or between ourselves. We didn't refer to or initiate conversations about our prior losses with others, including the Drs. When asked, we gave curt unemotional answers to their questions. If they wanted information, outside of what I felt was relevant to the current pregnancy with Bliss and Strycker, I simply and politely responded, "I don't believe that is relevant to my current pregnancy". If they began to pity me, I would quickly remind them, that the losses were behind me, and now my focus was on the current pregnancy.

You must live from the present in every thought and deed. Perfect health, has to be at your core and the foundation from which you are currently creating the life that you seek. If you are living from your past Dis-ease, you can only create more of the same. In everything you do, speak and exist from a place of who you desire to be, rather than who you were. In the moment you choose to come from a place of absolute perfect health, then what happened in the past, will no longer define who you are and what you are able to be.

> **Action Step:** Note when you have a physical expression of your energy. When does it occur? With whom does it occur? What steps can you take so that it does occur? What do you need to do to focus your energy on perfect fertility?

Tip# 7 - Stopped Using the Phrase "Trying" to Conceive:

I have completely dropped "try" from my vocabulary as it relates to having the things that I want in my life. It is a disempowering word that simply means, you are on the fence about what you want and your decision to go after what you want. Or worse, "try" means to attempt without succeeding. When you take out the word try, it immediately gives you power, and declares that you are clear and ready to take inspired action; that you have belief in yourself, and are ready to succeed. Sadly, yet honestly, if you are just "trying" to do something, chances are you won't actually get it done. Reflect upon your life to date, when you say try, is there a hidden truth, that you are giving yourself an out, however small? In my experience, when someone says, "Tiph, I'll try", they rarely if ever get it done.

I stopped "Trying to Conceive" and simply stated, I Will Conceive in the next few months. There was no equivocation or hesitation.

Be particularly mindful of how you refer or engage with other ladies, you are "TTC". Don't engage in that sort of talk. Don't for a second, speak the TTC aloud! You are officially IWC- I WILL CONCEIVE!

Tip# 8 - Stopped Frequenting Forums and Chat Rooms for the "infertile"—

"Do not listen to those who weep and complain,
for their disease is contagious."

Og Mandino

Certainly, this will rub many of you the wrong way. I get that. However, consider the following-

    a. We are the sum of the five closest people to us.

    b. We have to guard our thoughts and ALL negativity.

    c. We have to be mindful of our words

    d. We need to surround ourselves with those who have overcome.

    e. You are NOT infertile, so why are you hanging out there?

    f. See all of the previous pages!

As an illustration, here is a "profile signature" (profile details in a forum) from an infertility forum:

Me: 31 - PCOS
DH: 32 - Perfect
Married for 2 years trying to conceive the entire time
Parents to 2 rescue furbabies - Chey & Phoebe
2009 - TTC Naturally
2010 - OB/GYN
1st Clomid-50 unsupervised
  - No reaction
2010 - RE
2nd Clomid - 50 then upped to 100mg
  - No Reaction
2011 - Beginning of year we decide to take a break so DH can get a new job with some better insurance coverage
October/November 2011
IUI Cycle #1
Day 3-17- Gonal-F
Day 18 - Ovidrel trigger shot
Day 20 - IUI #1 (11/4/11)
3 HPTS all
11/18 - Beta - 22
11/20 - Beta- 26 declared non-viable.

Was that inspiring? Do you see how this person *IS* their Dis-Ease? Do you feel the hopelessness and frustration? This is not to suggest that she isn't a lovely person. However, this is merely to demonstrate, how the negativity can come in, even when wrapped in support and positivity.

There are other ways to get support in a more expansive, generative way. Here are a few ideas: (a) start a group of IWCs on Facebook or Twitter; (b) start a group on meet-up (c) create a blog of IWCs (d) put in ad in Craig's List. (e) Get a fertility coach, who spends 80% on mindset, 10% on dealing with the lingering physical effects of your stinking thinking, and 10% on support; (f) pull together so other liked minded women and go in together on a fertility coach group program. I know I personally host one via teleseminar. If you want more information on working with me directly, you can contact me at **Tiphanie@TheYayMe-University.com**. This is designed to defray some of the costs, as being fertility challenged, can cost a pretty penny/euro indeed.

The wonderful thing about the internet is that you are able to connect with people who are seeking what you are seeking. Remember, what you are seeking is always seeking you, you have to be prepared and have space to receive it! Just think, you are reading this book, right now and have the ability if you choose to connect with me further- this is NOT a coincidence.

Forums, though well intentioned, can also plant the seeds of doubts in your pregnancy. I can tell you, this absolutely happened with me. In one forum, I met a forum member, who was the "go to person" for information regarding IVF. Well, what I wasn't aware of at the time, was she was a bit of a drama queen, and had a lot of subtle negative energy around her. She often recounted her stories of miscarriages and wore them, like a badge of honor. For her, her miscarriages had become her identity and therefore made her an expert on IVF, and pregnancy loss. Not realizing this at the time, I conversed with her regularly, and I identified with her losses, experiencing at that time, 3 losses of my own.

Though well meaning, she was a negative person—you know, one of those people who always "hoped for the best but expected the worst", and disguised or couched her negativity in loving support. She mentioned to me in just about every heartfelt communication how she lost her babies and ALL the women who lost the babies had repeated miscarriages and the gestational ages of miscarriages. Worse, she made a point to tell me, that just because I was using IVF, didn't mean that the pregnancy itself would be any better. Now, she may not have even realized what she was doing by saying these things to me. In many ways, she was in fact quite helpful with the planning of the treatment, as we elected to do IVF in Europe rather than in America, where is way cheaper; but that is where her usefulness ended. Since I so identified with her, her failures were my failures. Her ANGLES and points of view, became my points of view; her possibilities became my possibilities. The thought of her losses after IVF played over in my mind like a broken record. Every day, I had the same thought, that I would lose my babies on the day of my baby shower/ going away party at the approximate gestational age she lost her IVF twins. I literally was "fighting" that thought, constantly. The more I resisted that thought, and stayed in communication with her, the more that thought grew. Also, since I was still in that negative toxic environment with my ex and family members, it was like vortex of negativity- unworthiness, negative seeds, dealing with toxic family members, the ex. In hindsight, it's no surprise that I lost those babies, the exact day that I feared I would- the day of my baby shower and in dramatic form. I literally, had to deliver on the babies in my truck on the way to the hospital. The thought was implemented in my subconsciousness by a woman who was also having fertility issues and a lot of fears around them. Those thoughts, played into my already negative thoughts, and the result, was lost babies- The exact day that I created in my mind, planted by a seed from a well-meaning, yet clueless member in a forum. I don't blame her, but I understand now, that when you are creating, you have to surround yourself with people who have had success; not those that are still caught in the vortex of desperation, fear, self-loathing, anger, confusion.

<hr>

Action Step: Are you a TTC forum frequenter? Do you have a profile signature? What does that profile signature say? What are the predominant conversations for which you engage in in the forums? Are you speaking things into being? Or are you in the "hope" and "baby dust" category? How can you make a different choose?

Tip# 8 - Said NO to Everything, Anything and Anyone, That Was NOT in Alignment with Getting Pregnant, Staying Pregnant and Delivering Healthy Babies—

"Success depends on getting good at saying no without feeling guilty. You cannot get ahead with your own goals if you are always saying yes to someone else's projects. You can only get ahead with your desired lifestyle if you are focused on the things that will produce that lifestyle."

Jack Canfield

So often we are taught that loving ourselves is selfish and that self-sacrifice is a good thing. I submit, that sacrifice is not all it's cracked up to be. So often in our culture, we are taught that sacrificing one-self is how we demonstrate love, compassion, and good character; after all, no one wants to be seen as "selfish", right? What I think is lost is the fact that sacrifice ultimately leads to regret, sadness, and other non-creative thoughts. *Sacrifice is defined by loss and deprivation*. When has deprivation and loss ever been associated with feeling good? What I have come to understand, is that you can never ever sacrifice your joy. When you sacrifice your joy you are saying several things:

(1) You are saying that there isn't enough, that there isn't abundance in the Universe, when we know that there is. If two thoughts cannot occupy the same space, then how could we on one hand, sacrifice ourselves because having what we desire would mean that someone would have to go without; while simultaneously believing that the Universe is abundant? Can you see the inherent contradiction?

(2) It also tells the Universe/God/Mother Earth/Spiritual Guide, that you are not enough; that there are others that are more deserving than you. We know that this sort of thinking is what has had us stuck in neutral for years. We are all deserving, but we are ALL RESPONSIBLE FOR OUR OWN CREATIONS!

(3) What good feeling can ultimately come from it? If you are believing that you have to sacrifice what you want, because

there isn't enough in the Universe, and/or you are unworthy. How are you possibly going to create new things from such negative beliefs and feelings? Learn to say no, to those things that require a "sacrifice", in the sense of deprivation. If you cannot give from your overflow and/or what you must give, is not in alignment with having your family, SAY NO! A price, any price that tells you that there is not enough, so you must give up your heart's desire is TOO HIGH!

Tip# 9 - Let Go of and Released the Babies I Lost.

"You can clutch the past so tightly to your chest that it leaves your arms too full to embrace the present."

Jan Glidewell

Through the law of attraction, I learned that two things cannot occupy the same space. Have you ever tried to have negative thoughts and be happy at the same time? It's simply not possible. The principle that two things can't occupy the same space was also true for my heart and my womb. By holding on to the feelings of "why me" and longing for the babies I lost, there was simply no room in my heart and body for new babies. While I attempted to remain "positive", my heart was longing for those babies, particularly the twins. In many ways, it was the way in which I lost them that was particularly traumatic. Also, I was so confused because by the time I was pregnant with the twins, I had already read the Secret, watched the movie, and was able to attract some awesome things to my life. Losing those babies, on the one day, that I was being "celebrated", in dramatic fashion (delivering one baby in the car), was so indicative of how I felt about myself at the time. I held on to the loss of the babies, because in a way, it "filled" me up. The search for answers, gave me something to do.

Also, remember that I didn't allow myself to feel the emotions and release them. Instead, we immediately hopped back on the IVF train, a few months later. In hindsight, I am not surprised it was a miserable failure. We were so messed up, and had NO business attempting to create. We were still so full of anger, confusion, lack of belief, it is a wonder we survived at all.

For those of you who have experienced the pain of miscarriage, you have to let go of what could have been. I am not saying that it won't ever sting to think about the losses. It absolutely will. In fact, when you successfully get pregnant, stay pregnant and deliver, it will actually sting a little more; the babies you then hold in your arms, will make you long to know the ones that are gone. This is perfectly normal, so don't beat yourself up. What I invite you to do, is let go of all of the expectations you had around the pregnancies you lost. Release the confusion, upset, rage, and "why ME's". I would even invite you to run some DE Way clearings, as discussed in The RADICAL Self-Expert book. Give yourself a date. Now, you are saying, you can't put a time limit on pain. I am telling you, YES YOU CAN! You are in control of your mind, you can choose something else. I didn't say it would be easy, but it is POSSIBLE. Allow yourself a final day of mourning, then let go and make the space in your heart and womb for your new viable pregnancy. You cannot bring forth life, when you are still longing and mourning death. Remember, two things cannot occupy the same space.

Tip #10 - Developed My Intuition Muscles.

Intuition can be cultivated and developed; in order to do this it must be recognized and appreciated; if the intuitive visitor is given a royal welcome when he comes, he will come again; the more cordial the welcome the more frequent his visits will become, but if he is ignored or neglected he will make his visits few and far apart.

Charles Haanel

I must admit that my intuition muscles were as weak as Alfalfa in the Little Rascals! I did not trust my inner voice at all! When you don't value yourself or believe yourself worthy, certainly, anything that originates with you, is deemed "untrustworthy". I ALWAYS sought the approval of others, and/or allowed their opinions to ultimately be my decisions. I trusted them, even when I knew, in every ounce of my being, that opinion and decision went against my desires, and most importantly my best interest. You must trust yourself.

Not trusting my intuition resulted in two of my lost angels between April of 2007 and November 2007. As discussed earlier in how unworthiness showed up, I did NOT trust my intuition. I knew that taking the medication BOTH times was NOT ok, yet I did it anyway. I didn't listen to my own voice. In both of those instances, I knew, based on my own research and inner knowing, that a medication, that was prescribed for me for a non-life threatening simple, readily treatable condition, could have waited until the second trimester to address. Still, after these losses, I didn't listen to myself.

Later, when I was pregnant with the Twin Angels, my well-meaning Dr., prescribed some invasive procedures for me, based upon "his determination" that I was "high risk". Here again, I relied on his assessment and opinions, rather than my own inner-knowing. Further, I witnessed some questionable hygiene practices by the ER physicians, and technicians and said nothing! For example, one doctor had put on a sterile glove and then grabbed his chair where God only knows how many bacteria was and then used the **same** glove for a vaginal exam. I was thinking at the time, he has been sitting there and God knows who else, he should change his glove, before doing this vaginal exam. Yet, I said NOTHING! I was weak, and didn't listen to my voice. Even though I wanted to scream, WHAT THE FUCK??? I stuffed down my intuition, my inner knowing and what I knew to be true for me. Ultimately, me not listening, resulted in an infection, to one of the Twin Angeles, and consequently, both Angeles had to be delivered prematurely. It is absolutely worth noting, that the pathology report, revealed that those Twin Angeles were PERFECT in every way. I must tell you, there is no pain, like the pain of delivering babies that you know will take one breathe and pass right before your eyes.

I share these losses with you, not to frighten you, but to tell you that YOU HAVE TO BE A RADICAL SELF-EXPERT. You have to take a stand for you, no one, can do that but YOU!

By the time I was pregnant with Bliss, Strycker and Spring, I was a RADICAL SELF EXPERT; Simply stated, I was the expert, everything else was just data. If it wasn't in line with what my inner knowing said, I wouldn't do it. If I saw a practice by one of the physicians, that was less that I deemed hygienically ok, I demanded they put on another set of gloves; if the sheet didn't look clean enough, I wouldn't sit on it. There were NO vaginal exams unless absolutely necessary and an external ultrasound was inconclusive. Now, many of you, may see this as extreme, but again, I knew what was right for me, and anything less was UNACCEPTABLE. You have to trust your inner knowing, your intuition. You are the authority and expert on YOU! The trick is to not cloud your intuition in negative thoughts or emotions. Your intuition is NOT fear or doubt based. It is strong and powerful.

"Listen to your intuition. It will tell you everything you need to know."
Anthony J. D'Angelo

Intuition comes very close to clairvoyance; it appears to be the extrasensory perception of reality"
Alexis Carrel

As previously mentioned, sabotage is ever so subtle at times. The obvious instances are of course, easier to manage, but the subtle acts of sabotage are ever so subtle, and those are the ones for which me must be on the lookout for. For those of you who have the complete unconditional, nothing but positive support of your friends and family, that is awesome. For many of us however, such is NOT the case. As with many of our goals in general, some are deemed "acceptable in the sight of our friends and families, others not so much. In fact, for some of your goals, you may find not only are they not supportive, but down right opposed to the idea, but they never directly say so. For example, in weight loss, after you decide that you want to get rid of a few extra pounds, she may offer to take you to the latest all you can eat pizza place, or offer you a piece of your favorite candy, saying, you can start your diet tomorrow. You as many others, are thinking, why? Why would someone who is my "friend" sabotage me? Well, several theories have been proffered, (1) they may have a vested interest in you not accomplishing the thing that you want; (2) what you want, may run counter to what they want, and they aren't even aware of it, and/or (3) they may not even be consciously aware they are sabotaging you.[vi]

Applying these ideas to your fertility- perhaps your friends and/or family members see you as having it all. For example, they great job, money, great romantic relationship, and they only thing you have not been able to achieve to date is becoming pregnant. Comparatively, they have none of the other successes, but can breed like a rabbit. You becoming pregnant, or by other means becoming a parent threatens the dynamic of your relationship. She needs to make herself feel better knowing, that she has the one thing that you could not achieve. Interestingly, it doesn't occur to her to go and accomplish the other successes, in career and education. She is just content with the fact that she has one up on you.

Another illustration would be in the case where you have a lot of childless friends and/or family members that fear that they will lose you if you become a parent. They have a clear interest in things remaining just as they are.

Note the things people say to you about your fertility. This will absolutely clue you as to whether there is some sabotage at play. More importantly, ask yourself how does it feel when the things are said. Here are some examples:

- ▶ "Maybe God doesn't want you to get pregnant." If it's God's will, you will have a baby."

- ▶ "I don't think assisted reproductive technologies is godly or appropriate. If you were supposed to have a baby, you would have one already."

- ▶ "You want to spend how much on IVF? I don't think I could give myself shots."

- ▶ "I did some research and the likelihood of IVF working is quite low. I read that a lot of women had to do more than 3 rounds of IVF before it worked. Why would you want to use someone else's sperm/eggs? What if they mix up your embryos at the clinic?"

- ▶ "Just keep praying and asking God and maybe you will get your baby. Maybe you should just give up and adopt. You already have a child(ren) why would you want more? Just love the ones you have already. At your age, why are you thinking of having a baby?"

- ▶ "Are you sure you want to do this? Well, I just want you to be happy, so if you are happy, I will support you."

These are but a few ways sabotage creeps in. Sadly, these people think they are being helpful and supportive.

> **Action Step**: Note what is being said to you and by whom. How does it feel? How will you choose to handle it?

Tip# 11 - Used Allies Often and Regularly

"You are the average of the five people you spend the most time with"

Jim Rohn

Being selective with who you share your dreams with is important. You want to select people who share your energy and have succeeded in overcoming their fertility challenges. This tip ties in with the other tips above. I relied heavily on two people during my pregnancy with Bliss and Strycker; these were my allies. They were the only two people with whom I shared my Dr.'s visits, and updates with. It is NOT an accident that one of the people, overcame her fertility challenges, and has a set of twins, and the other, had twin to twin transfusion syndrome and needed inter-utero surgery to save the life of her babies; Both of those women now how wonderful families. The thing is, with my first Ally, she went through IVF, succeeded on the first try, using many of the techniques I am sharing with you. Her presence reminded me that it is possible, to become pregnant and deliver healthy perfect babies, despite the odds. My second Ally reminded me that I create my reality, not a dr. When a Dr. told her, her babies would die, she said she, "F*&% that", and both of her babies are alive well and thriving. They provided me with inspiration, motivation and held the space for me, when I was not able to hold the space for myself. When I needed prayer, they didn't beg God for me, but were in agreement with me, about my heart's desires. They always spoke in the present tense about the babies, and recognized our individual power to create.

It will be a challenge for you to find the Allies that you need in a chat room/forum and the like, full of TTC'ers. How can they hold the space of belief and faith for you, when they can't hold it for themselves? They don't know what they don't know. If they knew what to do, they would be successful right now!

Other Subtle Sabotage Comments, Statements, Etc...

In addition to the language highlighted above, friends' and family members' sabotaging efforts, will show up in irrational and sometimes hostile criticism. Some things you may have heard or hear are:

> ▶ "You already have a good life, why can't you just be happy with that?" "You should just focus on the one you have." "Or, I would never use IVF, it is against nature."

They say these things, as if, somehow, you can't desire and/or have more for yourself; or because you have children, wanting more is somehow wrong?

Interestingly, these same people go to the Dr. for other ailments to remedy a problem, yet you are not permitted to seek a remedy for your fertility challenge, right? One of my other favorites, is, "the world is populated enough with children"- as if your child is going tip the scales to global famine? Please notice, how completely unfounded in logic these statements are.

While you cannot control others, you can control how you choose to respond to people. I just want you to be aware of the importance of your mindfulness to subtle sabotage.

Ally Checklist- Distinguish Allies from Subtle Saboteurs

1. Are they being encouraging and telling you to "go for it" or are they sending messages to keep things as they are?
2. What is their first reaction? Is it negative or positive?
3. Is the first thing spoken isn't negative.
4. How do you feel when you hear what they have to say?
5. Do they act in alignment with what you have specifically stated that you wanted?
6. Do you feel empowered by what is said?
7. Do they immediately begin the tidal waves of "how" questions?
8. Do their words cause a chain reaction of expansive thoughts, i.e., after their initial response, you feel good, and then your conversa-

tion turns to next steps to get what you desire... they are seeing and being possibilities for you.

9. Are their words, words of action? For example, you tell them you want to try IVF, and their next statement is, "let's find a Dr., or how can I help you, etc."
10. What is discussed is about you getting support, not about their feelings. For example, "What can I do to support you? How can I love you in this moment? What do you need/want from me right now?
11. Does it feel light or heavy to be in relationship with her?

Action Step: Find some Allies! If you were like me, where allies were few and far between, get a coach. I offer coaching, and have found, that it does make a difference. My heart certainly goes out to those women, who do not have support and I feel honored to support them in getting pregnant, staying pregnant and delivering.

Tip #12 - Created a Mantra:

A mantra is a sound, syllable, word, or group of words that is considered capable of "creating transformation.

Mantras are very important and assist you in remaining focused on your end result. As things show up in your reality, a mantra is a fun way to keep your energy high and creative. For example, when I was pregnant with Bliss and Strycker, I would always say" Healthy Babies, Healthy Babies, Healthy Babies". I would say this 3 times. Something so simple, kept me focused on the end result

Action Step: Create a mantra that reflects your end result. Make it easy and memorable and fun!

Tip #13 - Made a Creation/Request Box

"Ask and You Shall Receive" is one of the truths of the Universe. Although the principle of "Ask and You Shall Receive" is generally associated with a passage in the Bible, it is invariably a universal law. We ask a question to receive something, correct? Where in that passage or universal law does it say, "conclude to receive, or opine, or judge and receive"?

The mind is a computer, if you ask a disempowering question, it will search the hard drive for a disempowering answer.

Curiosity-consistently and continuously asking and living via empowering questions without necessarily going directly to the answer. The point of view, from which you ask the question, is a general sense of wonderment, a sort of surprise you are waiting to receive from the Universe. Curiosity is an energy that allows you to move from opinions, conclusions, assumptions, judgments, and points of views, to possibilities. It creates the space for you to be totally aware in any given moment, rather than somewhere locked in the past of what was and could have been.

NOTE: You don't have to consciously believe your empowering questions for them to be effective. Our minds are not designed to believe the questions, but rather, to seek answers to the questions posed it.

My creation box, was about me asking questions and allowing my energy to guide my "answers." Even when the answer showed up, I would ask another question. For example, one of the first questions I asked after losing the babies was, "What's it gonna take for me to get some freakin babies?" At that moment, in the shower, the answers started streaming to me like I was in the movie the matrix. I didn't stop asking questions though. Questions, create space and are infinitely more creative than affirmations. Ask and you shall receive is one of the truths of the universe. Every time I desired something, I would pose it in the form of a question and put it in my creation box. As, I was putting it in the creation box, I would literally be the energy of the thing I desired. I allowed myself to place my request with the universe, knowing it HAS to answer. It doesn't know good or bad, it just responds to our questions.

So check this out, if you ask questions like, "why can't I stay pregnant?" or "Why can she have babies and not me", have you noticed that the universe responds??? If it can respond to the things you don't want, it can respond to the things you want. Ask and you shall receive.

For me, a creation box, was about letting go in faith that what I desired was already here for me. Interestingly, I placed 3 baby names in my creation box, 3 years ago when I created it. When we delivered Bliss and Strycker, we were so thrilled and delighted to have them, we didn't even think about the other name in the box, or having another baby. Much to our surprise, 6 months after delivering Bliss and Strycker, we were pregnant with Spring! It just goes to show you, that the energy, questions and taking enlightened action, are powerful. While we didn't get triplets, we came pretty darn close!

Do not limit the amount of things you place in your box. The more things you put into your box, the more things via opportunities, people and information, will be delivered to match your ideals.

Tip #14 - Learned How to Pray and/or Connect to Source in a Way That was Empowering Rather than Punishing or Disempowering

"Most people do not pray; they only beg."

George Bernard Shaw

As a preacher's kid (PK) raised "in the church", we were taught to pray in a way, that was grounded in fear, desperation, disempowerment, and lack of faith. Ironically, we were also taught that "God is Love". I may be a little quirky, but when did fear, desperation, lack of faith and disempowerment, become loving? Call it God/Source/Mother Goddess/Spirit/Universe, whatever feels right to and for you, praying from a point of desperation or fear, is not based in faith and belief. I do believe in God, and what I understand now, is, God is not a punishing God. He does not withhold things, until you are worthy. God has given us a mind. As in Proverbs, "As a man thinketh, so he is". If you come from and think from fear and doubt, you will be fearful and riddled with uncertainty. Those two things will be remain obstacles in your life and show up in various ways, including yourself sabotage of opportunities.

If you are a prayer, when you pray, you ask, believe and receive. If you believe, you don't go and ask again and certainly don't beg. Don't see God as someone who is punishing. He wants for you, what you want for yourself, remember that!

"God gives us dreams a size too big so that we can grow in them."

Author Unknown

Here is an awesome excerpt from Napoleon Hill's Think and Grow Rich written in 1938. It speaks directly to how we should pray, and our approach to prayer.

"If you are an observing person, you must have noticed that most people resort to prayer ONLY after everything else has FAILED! Or else they pray by a ritual of meaningless words. And, because it is a fact that most people who pray, do so ONLY AFTER EVERYTHING ELSE HAS FAILED, they go to prayer with their minds filled with FEAR and DOUBT, which are the emotions the subconscious mind acts upon..."

Napoleon Hill[vii]

It is important to remember, that God is not punishing you, sentencing you to a life of unhappiness and infertility, because you made choices in your past, that weren't wise. The fact of the matter is, when you know better, you do better. When I used to think of the things I did in my past, trying to get someone to love me, and want me, I literally would cringe. What was true for me then, was I NEEDED love, and I would act from my subconscious thoughts that I was un-lovable, so I had to do things, to "get people to love me". Now, that I am a Radical Self Expert, when those feelings come up, I manage them. I recognize they aren't real or true, that it's old programming and replace those sabotaging thoughts, with some that are loving and creative. God is not punishing me; he loves me and wants for me, what I want for me. As noted by Albert Einstein, *"God may be subtle, but he isn't plain mean."*

When you pray, pray with confidence, that what you want for you, God wants for you. In fact, the best thing you can do as a believer, is to live the life of your dreams, and teach others, who now fear God and consequently refused to have a relationship with him, that there is another way. You can let your light shine brightly and be a testament, to a loving, forgiving, empowering God. Neale Donald Walsh, in his book, Conversations with God, noted:

"You cannot create a thing—not a thought, an object, an event—no experience of any kind—which is outside of God's plan. For God's plan is for you to create anything—everything—whatever you want."

Neale Donald Walsh

Tip# 15 - Did an Expansive Meditation Daily

"The kind of spirituality I value is one in which you get great joy out of contributing to life, not just sitting and meditating, although meditation is certainly valuable. But from the meditation, from the resulting consciousness, I would like to see people in action creating the world that they want to live in."

Marshall Rosenberg

As a certified Meditation Master, I know the power and importance of meditation. The benefits of quieting your mind and spirit are enormous, ranging from improved health, stress reduction, slowing the aging process to inner peace, self-love and improved relationship; The list of benefits run from A-Z and then some. Meditation though, was a great start, but I wanted to add some rocket fuel to it. I created and developed something called expansive meditation. It involved allowing me to expand out beyond my body. It allowed me to remember, that I am an infinite being and infinite possibilities are available to me. I am NOT limited by what lies to the left or right of me. Thoughts become things and allowing myself to go behind my subconscious mind's limitations, helped me to stumble on my miracle herb. It also allowed me to be in the space of creation and connect with the power of who I "BE" free from all the mind yuck. I didn't always know what to do next, or where to find a physician, product, or even where to live. We would make the decision on faith, believing that the next step would unfold for us when it was time. As the great Dr. Martin Luther King pointed out, *"Take the first step in faith. You don't have to see the whole staircase, just take the first step."* It is worth noting here, that I personally make a distinction between expansive meditation, visualization and "typical meditation". Visualization involves more the conscious guiding of my imagination; it is the intentional process of creating a mental picture, such that it creates a feeling of me being in that mental picture. When I visualize, I literally feel the feelings as if I were in the picture. I do not allow myself to make a distinction between what I am visualizing, and what is "reality". Meditation on the other hand, is more about relaxing, and calming you. Expansive meditation, as indicated above, is more about moving beyond your physical surroundings; a higher level of possibility and consciousness. I believe Albert Einstein put it best, *"Problems cannot be solved at the same level of awareness that created them."* *Albert Einstein*

Tip #16 - Active Visualization Daily

"When confronted with a situation that appears fragmented or impossible, step back, close your eyes, and envision perfection where you saw brokenness. Go to the inner place where there is no problem, and abide in the consciousness of well-being."

Alan Cohen

Visualization is a powerful way to get inside of the feeling of the babies being here. You have to see things in your mind before you can experience them in the outer world. Do not confuse visualization with daydreaming. Visualization involves a clear picture of what you are seeking, **AND** having the feelings of that thing right now. It is directed and controlled. When you are properly visualizing, there is no strain or effort in holding the thought, if you are straining, it creates an energy that suggests there is some adverse condition that must be fought against. What you want is a harmonious mental state.

Charles Haanel, discusses visualization in his famous book, The Master Key System:

"Visualization is the process of making mental images, and the image is the mold or model which will serve as a pattern from which your future will emerge. Make the pattern clear and make it beautiful; do not be afraid; make it grand; remember that no limitation can be placed upon you by anyone but yourself; you are not limited as to cost or material; draw on the Infinite for your supply, construct it in your imagination; it will have to be there before it will ever appear anywhere else.

…The inventor visualizes his idea in exactly the same manner, for instance, Nikola Tesla, he with the giant intellect, one of the greatest inventors of all ages, the man who has brought forth the most amazing realities, always visualizes his inventions before attempting to work them out. He did not rush to embody them in form and then spend his time in correcting defects. Having first built up the idea in his imagination, he held it there as a mental picture, to be reconstructed and improved by his thought. "In this way," he writes in the Electrical Experimenter. "I am enabled to rapidly develop and perfect a conception without touching anything. When I have gone so far as to embody in the invention every possible improvement I can think of, and see no fault anywhere, I put into concrete, the product of my brain. Invariably my devise works as I conceived it should; in twenty years there has not been a single exception."[viii]

This is actually quite fun. It will help you "get inside" your visualizations and feel wonderful. Talk about them in the present tense. We would lie in bed and Dutch would tell me, how he took Bliss and Strycker into the backyard to play and how much they had. He didn't speak in the future tense, for example, he didn't see, *when* the babies get here, I will take them in the yard; Rather, he got inside of the visualization and spoke of it in the present tense. I would so engage him, with questions in the present tense, about what games they played, what the children did. It was a real as possible for us. When we were "there" in our minds, it felt fantastic!

Tip #17 - Sought Out Success Stories Rather Than Be in Regular Communication with Those That Were Still "Struggling"

Rather than being jealous of them, I used their successes as reminders, that it is possible to have what I want, more babies! As I explained upon, one of them used IVF, and successfully delivered twins. The other, delivered a healthy baby, fell pregnant again with twins, but was faced with her twins having Twin-to-Twin Transfusion syndrome. She had to be hospitalized for about 2-3 months from what I can recall. When everyone told her, she would lose her babies, she didn't listen. Her resolve to birth healthy babies fueled my resolve. I saw her success, as my success. Rather than identifying with the people who struggle to conceive, I choose to identify with those who faced challenges in the eye, and kicked that challenge's ass.

Every time I felt my faith or believe wavering, I would lean on my two allies. When that was enough, or they were unavailable, I would go to the Secret website, and scour it for pregnancy success stories. There are hundreds of stories, of women who healed themselves and became pregnant, after 10-14 years of "infertility". If they could do it, so could I! I identified not with the struggle, but with the success.

You too, have to identify with success stories. I am not saying, only women that have become pregnant, but women who have become pregnant AND delivered healthy babies. You need to see yourself in them, and them in you.

This is also tricky in that, you want to identify with their successes, but not their conditions or dis-eases. Be very mindful, of their success and do not get into the details of whether they had bleeding, or how many embryos they implanted, etc. Just know they overcame what seemed impossible and know that if they did, so can you!

Make success for you the rule rather than the exception!

> **Action Step:** Seek Out Success Stories

Tip #18 - Did Not Complain About the Process, or Potential Symptoms

*"Instead of complaining that the rosebush is full of thorns,
be happy that the thorn bush has roses."*

Proverb

Complaining is a waste of energy. Your energy and attention need to be focused squarely on the end result.

I was sick as a dog with the estrogen, progesterone and prednisone I was taking to get pregnant, stay pregnant and deliver healthy babies. No, they weren't prescribed for me necessarily, but it was a decision I made- more on that later.

When you say, that you are willing to do anything to get pregnant, including, taking shots, supplements, medications, using donor eggs, whatever the case may be, DO NOT COMPLAIN! It is negative limiting energy and reeks of ingratitude. Don't complain about the weight you're gaining, or the extra couple of hairs on your face. Who cares if you are a bit nauseous or can't eat certain foods or smoke. It is only temporary. You can release extra weight, you can eat the foods again in a few months. It won't last always. There is an end, and the reward of having those babies is priceless.

Further, for those of you who have had a few miscarriages, don't complain about the morning sickness or dread it. Instead, be thankful for it. It is a clue that your body is doing exactly what it needs to do to bring forth life. My successful pregnancies were textbook. I had every system on the list, right down to the hemorrhoids and itchy skin. At one point, I was so ill, I had to take a nauseous medication prescribed for chemotherapy patients. Still, I never complained, I remained in gratitude for how obviously healthy my babies were. If I didn't throw up one day, I was thankful for that. During my successful pregnancies, I actually lost about 40 pounds, because I was not able to eat. If you can imagine with the last pregnancy with Spring, I was desperately Ill, and still had to take care of 6 month of twins, without help.

The key here, is don't dread the pain of delivery, stretch marks, being sick, throwing up. If you do, you are saying that you are NOT willing to do anything, and you don't want to be pregnant. These things in a lot of cases, go along with being pregnant. Welcome ALL of those things. Welcome, the big stomach, morning sickness. Be excited for all of those milestones and symptoms. The more things you are grateful for, the more things you will HAVE to be grateful for.

Tip #19 - Recognized that Doctors Were NOT Gods They are Human and Ultimately are Here to Serve Me, Not the Other Way Around.

"The best use of a physician's knowledge is to teach patients how to heal themselves."

Dr. David Simon

"Drugs are not always necessary. Belief in recovery always is".

Norman Cousins

"A Short History of Medicine

2000 B.C. - "Here, eat this root."

1000 B.C. - "That root is heathen, say this prayer."

1850 A.D. - "That prayer is superstition, drink this potion."

1940 A.D. - "That potion is snake oil, swallow this pill."

1985 A.D. - "That pill is ineffective, take this antibiotic."

2000 A.D. - "That antibiotic is artificial. Here, eat this root."

Author Unknown

The reality is, that you have to be a Self-Expert. You get information from the doctor, but it is just that, information. It doesn't mean he or she is right. You have to decide, if the information you receive, is something you want to act upon after consulting your intuition (gut) or not. I am so thankful for all the doctors, and the service they provided to us; however, they are just people, operating from their training. It would be wonderful to think, that the textbooks have encountered every single mutation, combination, and illness, ever known, but that simply isn't the case. Further, as great thinkers have observed, if you want to treat the disease, you have to treat the mind first.

I blindly, followed the doctor's opinions with the 5 losses, and it resulted in losses. I took medicine when I knew, it would not be wise for me to do so and against my gut; Exams were performed on me, because it was "customary", and I allowed it to happen. From those experiences, I had to learn that no one is more of an expert on me, than me! I know what my body is capable of, because I control the switchboard, MY MIND!

Your physician should be a partner in your fertility journey. With the losses, they were the drivers, and I was not even in the car, I was in the trunk. Where I succeeded, I consulted with them, but ultimately told them, what my course of treatment was to consist of. I choose to use herbal supplements, I choose to use progesterone and prednisone, and the like. There was this inner knowing, that all was well, and I was exactly where I needed to be. Doubt or hesitation as to my course of treatment, rarely entered my mind- if/when it did, I would go to my quiet place, and listen for the answer. The answer always came, ALWAYS! Then I would follow that answer with another question- "How does it get even better?"

Remember, when you are selecting a physician to assist you in your journey, choose a partner. If you find that he/she is telling you what to do, rather than consulting with you, then GET ANOHER physician. You and your physician must be aligned as any resistance, will only feed fear and doubt. There has to be a trust in yourself that extends outward to him-not the other way around. You don't trust him first, and then follow. You trust you first, and then receive the information. Remember, partnership, not dictatorship!

Tip #20 - Was Ok When People Disagree with Me.

"To go against the dominant thinking of your friends, of most of the people you see every day, is perhaps the most difficult act of heroism you can perform."

Theodore H. White

I too, was one of those people who feared discourse and disagreement. As a result of not trusting myself, and not knowing my value and worth, the opinions of others meant more to me than my own. Here again, we are back to the DECISION of doing what it takes to have babies. When you make a decision, you have to be courageous and focused enough to withstand, whatever comes your way. The awesome thing is, it will show you, who you are energetically aligned with, and who your saboteurs are. For example, some people may disagree with you taking the natural route, or using acupuncture, IVF, a surrogate, a particular doctor. The reality is, people have something to say about any and everything. Your job is simply not to receive the information as "true" when it isn't. Consult your Allies, but ultimately, be a Radical Self-Expert; be ok with being different. Love yourself enough to trust you above all others. If other people don't agree, that is about them, not you. Just DO YOU!

Tip #21 - Questioned Everything I was Being Told.

"Trust yourself, then you will know how to live."
Johann Wolfgang von Goethe

I always checked in with myself, and if it didn't resonant, I didn't do it. For some reason, the person that questions things, is considered a nuisance. When you are a Radical Self Expert, gather the information, run it past your intuition and see, if it "feels" true for you or not. When a doctor tells you, he thinks you should use a medication, ask why? Ask can it wait? Ask questions! You DO NOT have to blindly accept things as true. I didn't question the doctors about taking a medication, and I lost 3 babies; didn't question the invasive procedures, lost 2 more babies. You are the authority on you. Gather data, notice I didn't refer to them as facts or data. They aren't facts, just data- hear it, and see what feels true for you.

Another example would be the use of red raspberry leaves. While it is commonly used for infertility and is considered a "uterine tonic", I questioned whether taking it would be right for me. For you see, in order to "tone" something, it has to be used, right? If you want to quiet the uterus to allow your embryo to implant, via natural or ART methods, wouldn't it make sense to want the uterus as calm as possible? Particularly in my case, where I had a history of repeated losses. The last thing I wanted my uterus to do was to contract and "tone". I wanted it supple and quiet to allow the babies to implant. Now certainly, some light cramping is normal, as it may signal the embryo is burying in. However, adding something that is said to contract the uterus is not a wise choice for me. Think about this, there is a reason why they tell women to take red raspberry leaf during the last weeks of pregnancy. It will help aid labor. For those of us with a history of miscarriage, aid in labor is the last thing we want until at least week 36 of our pregnancy.

When you hear information, imagine it is a coat and put the coat on your body. How does that coat feel? Do you feel light or heavy? Do you feel bolder, braver, are you standing more erect? Are you feeling powerful and an immediate sense of relief and "lightness"? If so, the information is more likely true for you. If you feel heavy and weighted down by it, chances are, it is not true for you. Now, when using this technique you must be mindful, that sometimes, based on our conditioning, something may feel heavy then light or light then heavy or a combination of the two. When this is the case, you have to go to what you desire; in this case a baby, and say, which information is more in line with what I desire, then take action based upon that.

William James says it so wonderfully, *"Seek out that particular mental attribute which makes you feel most deeply and vitally alive, along with which comes the inner voice which says, 'This is the real me,' and when you have found that attitude, follow it."*

Fertile Body...The Body Stuff...

"There is a revolution taking form that is significantly influencing how the Western medical community views health and disease. I have lectured and written countless books about the important role of perception and awareness in health and longevity–how awareness can actually transform matter, create an entirely new body. Our bio-chemical messengers act with intelligence (<u>innate wisdom</u>) by communicating information, orchestrating a vast complex of conscious and unconscious activities at any one moment. This "information transfer" takes place over a network "<u>linking</u>" all of our systems and organs, engaging all of our molecules of emotion, as the means of communication. What we see is an image of a "mobile brain: – one that moves throughout your entire body, located in all places at once and not just in the head. This body wide information network is ever changing and dynamic, infinitely flexible. It is one gigantic loop, directing and admitting information simultaneously, intelligently guiding what we call life."

Dr. Deepak Chopra MD

Many of you, probably purchased the book thinking, that I was only going to talk about supplements, acupuncture, and some sort of shortcut to a baby. I gave you all the tools to control the switchboard of your body, YOUR MIND; so you can instantly shift your thinking and have the things you so desire.

In order to be pregnant in the body, you must first be pregnant in the mind. Think about it this way, if I did not make the decision, take action, clear my history, and be open to the possibilities, I would NEVER have learned of the supplements, and other tools to become pregnant. Had I been stuck in the traditional way of thinking, I could not have used my intuition to find various supplements and become a Radical Self-Expert, in charge of my care. I would still be that weak timid victim, that listened to doctors, didn't listen to myself and still miscarrying and struggling to get pregnant.

There is absolutely a connection between the mind and body in wellness. Unquestionably, everything changed for me, the moment I shifted to a Radical Self-Expert mindset.

Tip#22 - Dutch Stopped Carrying His Cell Phone in His Pocket and Stopped Placing His Laptop on His Lap

There was a study done which revealed the connection between electromagnetic waves and the killing of sperm. Accordingly, Dutch no longer carried his cell phone in his pocket.[ix]

Tip#23 - Used Acupuncture Based On the Fertility Protocol[x]

I am the ultimate needle-phobe; if there was a show, on Extreme Needle phobias, you would see me front and center. However, again, we made the decision to do whatever it took to become pregnant. Acupuncture has been used extensively to treat a number of conditions from weight loss and Tinnitus to infertility and miscarriage. Derived from China, acupuncture has been used to successfully treat and in some instances reverse infertility for centuries. According to Dr. Gary Hull, the first published account in medical literature, dates back to 11 A.D. In brief, acupuncture analyzes 5 principal organs - the liver, spleen, heart, lung, and kidney. It is believed that the energy or "chi" may be blocked from these systems. Acupuncture seeks to restore the chi thereby bringing the body in balance and health. Promoting fertility is one of the many benefits of acupuncture. Acupuncture to kidney points releases psychological blocks that interfere with reproduction[xi]. Over the years, many healers and holistic health practitioners have recognized the efficacy of acupuncture. There are specific protocols that have been developed for various forms of fertility. For example, there are IVF protocols, fsh protocols, follicle protocols, hormonal protocols, and so on. Please see the appendix the exact protocol that we used. Also, we did an oracle protocol for fertility in Europe.

I had two acupuncturists, one in Southern California and one in Europe. The acupuncturist in Southern California was such a gift to us. She had a practice that she shares with her life partner. Dutch was treated as well as me. After a thorough examination, she determined that I was suffering from a spleen chi deficiency and Dutch a kidney chi deficiency. Accordingly, we were prescribed various foods and associated protocols to balance our respective chis; this was in addition to the fertility acupuncture protocol. They also provided for us, a list of supplements and information regarding miscarriage prevent and support for the sperm. The list of supplements discussed below and the acupuncture protocol, is attached in the appendix. Keep in mind; these supplements were prescribed after a personal and detailed examination. If you decide to seek an acupuncturist, some guidelines are:

(a) Make sure the acupuncture is specifically familiar with the fertility protocol. You don't want a generalist. The fertility protocol is very specific and based upon industry accepted research.[xii] Their specific expertise in the area of fertility is vital, because certain acupuncture points on the body are contraindicated after embryo transfer with IVF. You need to have a certified acupuncturist who is up to date on the specifics of fertility.

(b) Ask for fertility patient referrals- women and/or men that are willing to speak with you about their experiences with infertility and acupuncture

(c) Ask about their training, certification and state/government licensure.

(d) If you don't get a good "vibe" from the acupuncturist, LEAVE!

(e) Make sure communication is clear. My acupuncturist in California, was a native English speaker. My European acupuncturists, were not native English speakers, and spoke Dutch's native language of Dutch, German, and worked extensively with local fertility clinics.

(f) Make sure from the initial consultation, that all safety precautions are taken- disposable needles, clean environments, etc.

Tip #24 - No Caffeine

For a caffeine head like me, I LOVE TEA with creamer and splenda, going cold turkey was literally painful. However, I wanted to ensure that my body was in optimal condition for nourishing those babies. Dutch also eased up on the caffeine to ensure there was no further sperm DNA fragmentation.

Tip# 25 - No Sex and/or Orgasms for Me

We did not have intercourse, as we decided we didn't want anything "foreign" into the vagina that could in any way affect the cervix. Also, I was inserting progesterone tablets, and well, that would just be messy.

Also, orgasms contract the uterus, and that was NOT what I wanted to do. I wanted to quiet my uterus to allow it to nourish the babies.

Tip#26 Took Prescription Strength Progesterone, Baby Aspirin and Low-dose Prednisone[xiii]

Although there are extensive studies that support the efficacy of progesterone, aspirin and prednisone for idiopathic miscarriages. I used all three until 14 weeks. With the progesterone, I took, utrogestan and after the 12 week, tapered off. My progesterone was prescription strength, prometrium or utrogestan as it is known in Europe. Rather than take it orally, I used it vaginally, 200 mg per day, 3 times per day.

With the baby aspirin, I quit cold turkey at week 12. The protocol for idiopathic miscarriages, recommended baby aspirin until the second trimester.

Prednisone is a steroid, used to suppress the immune system to allow the embryo to successfully implant, without being attacked as a "foreign object". After extensive testing with the prior miscarriages, I had no immunological issues, or was ever diagnosed with the conditions associated with prednisone use in fertility. However, I decided that it was best after reviewing the study above and informed my doctor of my intention to take prednisone. I didn't quit taking prednisone cold turkey; it is definitely something to be weaned off. By the 14th week, I was no longer using prednisone at all. Initially, I was prescribed 5mg per day, which was cut in half to 2.5mgs, again stopping at the 14th week.

The "goal" as I understood it with prednisone, is to suppress the immune system to allow the embryo to implant without rejection. There is still considerable debate surrounding whether this is advisable, however, in Europe, is not uncommon for habitual miscarriages. A link for the study is included in the footnotes and reference section of this book.

Tip #27 - No Diet or Excessive Exercise

Dramatic diets and exercise may affect hormones, and since our since hormones are the heart of infertility, I wanted to keep them steady.

Tip #28 - Viburnum Prunifolium Black Haw[xiv]- Or, As I Call it, MY MIRACLE Herb!

Black Haw has quite an interesting story. Although the plant was used in the early 1800s as a home remedy, the first published account of the herb was in 1857. Dr. John King, an American family physician described the herb as a "uterine tonic". At that time, Doctors regularly and routinely prescribed it to prevent miscarriage or threatened abortion and also recommended it as a natural treatment for menstrual cramps and the after-pains of childbirth. From 1882 to 1926, (now omitted), the plant was officially listed in the United States Pharmacopeia from 1882 to 1926. In 1886, the herb was introduced into the National Formulary as an herbal antispasmodic and sedative.

Quite familiar with the herb, the Native Americans didn't reveal to early settlers the enormous benefits of "Black Haw". . Much of what was learned about Black Haw, came directly from Dr. King's Dispensatory medical and herbal textbook of 1854. According to Dr. King's text, Black Haw was good for boosting fertility and to preclude abortion.

An interesting though sad relic of American history, is the significant accounts of slave-owners forcing their pregnant slaves to eat black haw plants and berries, to prevent the slaves from terminating their pregnancies and ensuring a larger workforce. During slavery, slaves would take the powerful abortive agent *cotton root*, so as not have any children born into slavery or sold away from them later. Slaver owners in response, began widely using Black Haw. It is said, that the use of Black Haw was powerful enough to in fact, counteract the effects of cotton root [an abortive agent) taken with criminal intent. The use of Black Haw, enables the system to resist the deleterious influence of drugs so often used for the purpose of producing abortions

In addition to being used as a uterine tonic, Black haw is beneficial in the treatment of other health problems, including, menstrual cramps, false labor, asthma, nervous irritation, muscle spasms, easing symptoms of menopause, calming uterine muscles, morning sickness colic, lowering blood pressure, bronchitis and other lung diseases.[xv]

Evidence suggests, that scopoletin, which is the active ingredient that aides in muscle relaxation and in specifically in this case, the uterus. In 1866 Dr. E.W Jenks of Detroit described Black Haw as particularly valuable in preventing abortion and miscarriage, whether habitual or otherwise, whether threatened from accidental cause, or criminal drugging.

Dr. Macfie Campbell, and Dr. Leith Napier in the January 1885 reported at the British Medical Association, the effectiveness of Viburnum Profilium, aka Black Haw, in the Liverpool Chirgucal Journal, *"I have never seen ill consequences follow the administration of the medicine, however often the dose has been repeated. In two cases only has it been followed by slight headache. One patient inquired if she had not been taking quinine. The symptoms had been relieved; therefore it was not continued. In the other case, the patient had taken four grains of the extract every two hours. The only change was to extend the interval to four hours, and I then gradually discontinue it. Some patients have taken viburnum at intervals during the whole course of their pregnancy. It seems to act as an uterine tonic and sedative, and to relieve the woman of those harassing nervous forebodings which often lead to abortion. The patient, after taking only a few doses, has quite a changed expression. From a drawn, desponding look, her countenance becomes cheerful and happy. Since I have prescribed viburnum, it has not been necessary to keep the women in the horizontal position more than a few days; whereas, under the old treatment, they occasionally spent weeks in Led, and, after all, abortion has taken place. On some of the plantations in America, it is the popular belief a woman cannot abort if she be under the influence of* *black haw, although she may be taking medicine with a criminal intent. My experience would go far to confirm that opinion, for I have had patients in whom a succession of abortions have taken place, but, when under the influence of the medicine, they have been able to resist the severest tests-frights, falls, strains, etc.-and no ill effects have followed. With regard to the model of administering the drug: at first, the liquid extract was or(dared, but the smell was so strong, and objectionable, that the whole house became impregnated ; and in two cases,where the stomach could not retain it, the liquid was given as anenema.*[xvi]

Although safe for use during pregnancy to prevent miscarriage, it's use is not recommended by those with a history of liver and/or kidney problems and its use may produce gastrointestinal upset. Also, if someone has an aspirin allergy, they will unfortunately be **unable** to use Black Haw as it contains, contains salicin, a chemical relative of aspirin.[xvii]

This herb was too important to merely order online. Unfortunately, we weren't aware of its existence until after we arrived in Europe and did some extensive research. Dutch was able to locate an organic farmer in the northern part of the Netherlands close to the sea. When we inquired of the man (I affectionately refer to as "the Great Mad Scientist"), he was quite familiar with the herb. We drove up to the farm, and was able to purchase the tincture, which we watched him prepare. I am sure you can purchase this herb on the internet somewhere, however, I want to be clear, I did not purchase mine from the internet. For those of you, who may not be aware, many European countries, are quite heavily regulated in comparison to what we have come to expect in the United States. If a farmer, calls himself "100% organic" in the Netherlands, there is a government agency who darn well, will make sure that the farm is 100% organic. Just because it may not be a "drug" as defined by our Federal Drug Administration, in the Netherlands, that does not exempt them from a standard of care and honesty. I am so thankful to the Great Mad Scientist and his Family. They were absolutely wonderful to and for us! I used his herbs for both successful pregnancies. The herbs worked so well in fact, that Bliss and Strycker had to be induced and Spring was only 3 days early. Coming from 5 losses to have to crank up the Pitocin with Bliss and Strycker was and remains a gift indeed. If you would like more information on the Black Haw, just email me at **Tiphanie@ TheBookonPregnancyAfterLoss.com**. I would also add, my blood pressure was PERFECT throughout both pregnancies. Typically, in twin pregnancies, high blood pressure is a concern. Not in my case. It was consistently normal, and often commented on by my physician.

Tip #29 - Vitamin and Herbal Supplement Protocols Provided to Us by Our Licensed Acupuncturist in California

Here is the list of the supplements we took to get pregnant, stay pregnant and deliver healthy babies.

A. Calcium, Magnesium and Zinc-

I choose to take a supplement that contained all three, as the balance between the minerals is important. Rather, than trying to figure it out myself, I selected one, which contained the proper ration of Calcium: Magnesium: Zinc ratio.

▶ Calcium decreases high blood pressure, and increases blood flow to other muscles, including the reproductive organs. Calcium plays a part in insulin secretions from the pancreas. Insulin imbalance can lead to menstrual problems in women and lower sperm quality in men.

▶ Magnesium - Magnesium supports heart health, and helps to regulate heart beat and rhythm, which pumps blood to the whole body and the reproductive organs. Magnesium also plays a role in carbohydrate metabolism, and helps to regulate insulin via the pancreas; thereby reducing infertility by regulating blood glucose levels. Magnesium also helps to relax muscles, and even the reproductive muscles, thereby increasing your chances of fertility. Magnesium plays a vital role in muscle health. When there is a lack of magnesium in the muscle, spasms form, which can create painful P.M.S and menstrual cramping.[xviii]

▶ Zinc plays an important role in reproductive health. Follicular fluid level maintenance- low fluid levels in the follicles, the egg can't travel through the fallopian tubes to the uterus for implantation.

✓ **Hormone regulation:** zinc is one of a number of minerals that the body uses to for hormone level maintenance i.e. progesterone, testosterone and estrogen. Hormone regulation is particularly important during the 2nd and 4th stage of a female cycle. It is especially important during stage 2 and 4 of a woman's cycle.

✓ **Egg production:** Amounts of zinc are needed to produce mature eggs that are ripe for fertilization by the sperm.

✓ Equally importantly, according to The Centers for Disease Control's Assisted Reproductive Technology Report, low levels of zinc have been linked to miscarriages in early stage pregnancy.

B. Deep See Fish Oil 2400mg 2 times per day (mercury free).

C. Prenatal vitamin with less than 30% vitamin E

D. Bee pollen, Bee Propolis and Royal Jelly- (If you are allergic, don't take this!)

Mentioned in such religious books as the Bible, Talmud, the Koran, and the Book of Mormon, bee pollen has be used to treat various conditions dating back to the ancient scrolls of the far east. The benefits of bee pollen have been touted by the Egyptians, Romans and Greeks alike.[xix] It has been said, that bee pollen is a super-food because it is one of the most nutritious foods on the planet. Hippocrates (460 – 377 B.C.), was the first physician to focus on preventing disease with bee pollen as well as treating diseases.

Among countless other non-fertility related benefits, Bee Pollen helps to balance the hormone levels, increase libido, reduce inflammation in the reproductive organs, increase immune system and maintain egg health i.e. egg quality.

The specific amino acids, proteins, lips and nutrients inside of bee pollen and royal jelly, seem to boost the quality of some women's eggs. Given that royal jelly is used to help the queen bee produce, it is unsurprising, that it would be useful for fertility.

For those of you using IVF to create your family, bee pollen/royal jelly supplementation may help to improve the number and quality of your eggs. We used bee pollen prior to our attempt at IVF and it was successful, though we lost the babies later. Later when we tried IVF and failed we have over 13 eggs, many of which went to blastocysts.

Following the birth of Bliss and Strycker, I continued to use bee pollen for non-fertility related purposes, and was pregnant with Spring, less than 6 months after giving birth to Bliss and Strycker.

If you intend to use ART to create your family, begin using bee pollen/propolis at least 3 months before you begin treatments.

- ▶ **Royal Jelly** is the food of the Queen Bee. She lives approximately 6 years exclusively on royal jelly while the worker bees each honey and pollen and have a life span of 6 weeks.

- ▶ **Propolis** is a sort of natural antibiotic. It is a substance made by the honeybee, which protects again fungi, viruses and harmful bacteria. Additionally, propolis acts as a local anesthetic, reducing spasms, healing gastric ulcers, and strengthening capillaries.

E. Green Plus - Once I became pregnant, I no longer used green tea, because it contains caffeine.

F. Along with the prenatal vitamin, take an additional 800mcg of Folic Acid, also known as Folate. Folic acid is one of the best known vitamins essential for a healthy pregnancy and baby. Folate commonly known as folic acid is a B vitamin, which if taken before pregnancy and in the first few weeks of the first trimester, helps to prevent neural tube defects, congenital heart defects cleft palates, limb defects and urinary tract defects in developing fetuses. A deficiency may result is preterm labor, low birth weight, and fetal growth retardation.[xx] Some studies also suggest that a deficiency of folate, may increase the homocysteine level in the blood, which could potentially lead to spontaneous miscarriage and other pregnancy complications, such as pre-eclampsia and placental abruption.

G. Vitamin C[xxi] - Has been shown to improve hormone levels and increase fertility in women with luteal phase defect, according to a study published in "Fertility and Sterility". [xxii]

Dutch's Supplements and Protocol

The supplements prescribed for Dutch were quite extensive. **Free radicals** (which float around the body and damage other cells) have been said to be responsible for 40 sperm of sperm damage and DNA fragmentation. Thankfully, free radicals can be fought with antioxidants, vitamin A (beta-carotene), C, E, selenium and zinc.[xiii] Studies have now shown that damage to a man's sperm, may also result in either birth effects or miscarriages as well. The goal, of his supplements as explained to us, was to protect his sperm, from free radical damage, to limit any potential for DNA fragmentation.

His list consisted of:

1. **Pycnogenol** 125 milligrams per day for sperm morphology[xxiv] According to a study conducted by Dr. Scott Roseff, author of the study and Director of the West Essex Center for Advanced Reproductive Endocrinology, *"Up to 60% of infertile couples have difficulty conceiving due to abnormalities in the male's sperm. By taking Pycnogenol(r) to increase normally functioning sperm naturally, couples may be able to (or potentially) avoid in-vitro fertilization and either enjoy improved natural fertility or undergo less invasive and less expensive fertility-promoting procedures."[xxv]*

2. **L-Arginine** 2-4 g per day- L-Arginine has been shown to double semen volume and sperm health. "Effects of L-Arginine on Sperm." *L-Arginine Guide*. <http://l-arginineguide.com/effects-of-l-arginine-on-sperm.html

3. **L-Carnitine** 1,000- 12000 mgs per day- L-Carnitine is an amino acid which is essential for sperm cells to function properly. Both the quality and motility of sperm is improved with L-Carnitine.[xxvi]

4. **Zinc 60** milligrams per day-Zinc can be found naturally in foods, which aides in the metabolism of cells. It stimulates the important sperm enzymes and helps in the production of testosterone. A study concluded that a zinc deficiency

produces weak and malformed sperm. Another study determined that a zinc deficiency may be an important risk factor for low quality sperm and idiopathic (unexplained) infertility. "Semen is normally rich in zinc. Administration of exogenous systemic zinc to males with zinc deficiency can improve sperm production. Zinc sulphate therapy for infertile males with or without varicocelectomy may be an effective treatment."[xxvii]

The awesome news, is that where zinc is supplemented, testosterone and sperm count levels may be restored to acceptable levels "Zinc, B Vitamins (B6, B12 and folic acid), Vitamin C, and Antioxidants" for treatment of oligozoospermia, and found that they "are critical nutrients in the male reproductive system for proper hormone metabolism, sperm formation and motility."[xxviii]

Research suggests that daily consumption of folate (folic acid) and zinc can increase sperm count in subfertile men.[xxix] In a trial involving 14 men, zinc was administered over four months. The results of the study showed significant improvement in sperm count, in particular number of advanced motile and normal spermatozoa, and acid phosphates activity. Three wives of patients conceived.[xxx]

The benefits of zinc on sperm count have been documented in several studies involving idiopathic infertile men. Improvement with the administration of oral administration was significant.[xxxi]

5. **Vitamin A** - Beta Carotene 100,000 IU per day Vitamins A (beta carotene) is a fat-soluble vitamin and antioxidant that plays a key role in repairing damage caused by the environment and aging - and in preventing cellular damage due to oxidizing free radicals. As with the other antioxidants vitamin A improves sperm quality.[xxxii]

6. **Grapeseed Extract** - Grapeseed extract is a plant substance that that is said to be more powerful warding off free radicals than vitamin c, e and beta carotene. It provides a concentrated source of oligomeric proanthocyanidins.[xxxiii]

7. **Vitamin E** 800 IU per day- Vitamin E is an antioxidant which helps to improve both the quality and motility of sperm.

It is one of the vitamins, categorized as an "anti-oxidants", that are help to fight the free radicals discussed above reducing dna defects and fragmentation of the sperm. DNA fragmentation has been shown to greatly contribute to miscarriages and/or birth defects. Studies have shown that men who increase their intake of vitamin E, have improved sperm quality and motility, resulting in patients with an increased intake of vitamin E that have sperm quality or motility issues have improved their chances conceiving a baby by 10% after getting a few months of vitamin E supplements.[xxxiv]

8. **Vitamin C** 2,000 milligrams per day -For men, vitamin C has been show to protect sperm from free radical damage, which helps to reduce the change of miscarriage and chromosomal problems. It also appears, that supplemental vitamin C lessens the likelihood of the sperm clumping, thus making them more motile.[xxxv]

9. **Vitamin D** - Vitamin D has been determined to be positively associated with sperm motility.[xxxvi]

10. **CoQ10** - Coenzyme Q-10 (CoQ10) is an anti-oxidant found in seminal plasma and fluid. Several studies have concluded that there is a close correlation between CoQ10 levels and sperm count. Research indicates that there is improved sperm density and motility with CoQ10 supplementation. Equally importantly, research indicates that supplementation increases sperm morphology.

11. **Selenium** - Selenium is an antioxidant that protects both sperm and eggs from free radical damage. Free radicals can chromosomal damage in the eggs and sperm, leading potentially to miscarriages and birth defects. Further, selenium is necessary for the production of testosterone. Low selenium levels, affect sperm motility, because of the tail of the sperm being weakened and/or deformed.

12. **Calcium & Magnesium** - In 2001, a study concluded that calcium plays a vital role in spermatogenesis and fertility. One study determined that there was a positive correlation between calcium and sperm motility, linear motile sperm motility (LMSM), straight line velocity (VSL), curvilinear velocity

(VCL), mean angle of deviation (MAD), active sperm density (ASD), average path velocity (VAP) and lateral head amplitude (ALH).[xxxvii]

13. **Copper** - Copper is an essential trace element found, literally, in every cell in the body. Also, a powerful free radical fighter, copper is important in spermatogenesis.[xxxviii]

Diet:

We were instructed to eat organically as much as possible and also apply the diets prescribed for our respective chi deficiencies. Our chi deficiencies were diagnosed by our Licensed Certified Acupuncturists.

Conclusion

The last 5 years, have been the best and worst times of my life. My intention through this medium is to share my experiences, to show you what is possible when you are open to different ways of being and thinking, make a Decision, Become a Radical Self Expert and Believe in the possibilities. You may not get there, the way, you design, but you can get there! I am proof that it is possible. By all accounts, with every loss the odds were swinging against me, yet, I decided, believed and became an expert in me. You can do this too. I will not tell you, it will be easy, I will tell you however, that whatever you come up against, if you push through and know your truth, you can have, be and do anything you desire.

Mindset is about more than "positive thinking" and vision boards. You and your partner (if applicable), have to patch up the emotional and psychological cracks in your fertility. By doing so, you are making the space to receive all the tools you will need to make it possible. It is no accident that you read this point, it is no accident, that I am sharing my experiences with you right now. You sought answers, and now you have some. Perhaps this is all you will need, or just another piece of your puzzle. Be Open, make the Decision, become a Radical Expert, and Believe, and watch the magic of life unfold before you.

If you would like to connect with me further, it would be my absolute pleasure and honor. I am on Facebook at Facebook.com/TheYayMe-University, or on Twitter @ twitter.com/TiphanieJamVan, YouTube at TiphanieJVD.

Please visit my website **http://TheYAYMeUniversity.com** for more information on how you can become a Radical Self Expert, sign up for some awesome free goodies. Get your free 7 part video presentation of The RADICAL Self-Expert Method at **http://TheRADICAL-SelfExpertMethod.com**.

Warmly with Loads of YAY!

Tiphanie

Acknowledgments

Where do I begin? I haven't experienced true love from a lot of people in my life, but I have experienced TONS of Love from a few people… Growing up the way I did, I had no idea what love was. All I knew was I didn't want to be me. Some people have come into my life that showed me, that being me was all they wanted and needed. I am so Blessed.

To My Angels: Not a day goes by that I don't think about you. I know you are watching over Bliss, Strycker and Spring and I am grateful that you are their protectors.

To The Royals- Bliss, Strycker and Spring- You are PURE Joy. I still can't believe you are mine and I get to keep you. I am sooo in love with you. I finally know what it's like to experience pure unadulterated love. Your kisses and hugs are better than Crème Brule [heaven on a plate]! I love you beyond the stars, past the moon, around the world and back again. You are the most beautiful things I have ever seen, held, touched or experienced. What else is possible?

To Frederik VanDerLugt AKA "Dutch" AKA "Erik"- You have given me the most awesome gifts ever- Bliss, Strycker and Spring. We have literally been around the world and back again to get the beautiful gifts "from the sky". Thank you, thank you, and thank you. There are no words to express how truly grateful I am for those Blessings and the role you played in manifesting them. My heart is full and ever expanding. YAY!

To Guadalupe Ruiz Argleben AKA Farnsworth- What can I say? I love you beyond the moon. From the moment you walked in my office, I was your T-Diddy and You were my Farnsworth and I have been Blessed ever since. You have ALWAYS been true to me. Diddy and Farnsworth… Always and Forever [Napoleon Dynamite voice]. You always let me know that I was enough and then some. When the "fam" was mean to me, you became my "fam". Thank you! Thank you! Through all of those losses, you kept loving me and telling me I deserved babies, that I deserved love and that God loved me. When it seemed that no one in the world loved me, YOU DID! You always filled the gap and held the space for what could be possible. I am sooo proud of you and it fills my heart to love you. You are my Diddy of Motherhood! You rock on sooo many levels. I know that God loves me, because he allowed me to experience your love. Thank you for being my Ally, thank you for always choosing to love me. I VALUE YOU!

F.R.E.D - Thank you for stepping in when I was hurting so badly. You were the first person to show that "acting out" was not in my best interest. You lovingly, called me out, and then got me help at your expense. As I moved through the after effects of my childhood traumas and crazy choices, you were there seeing beyond the madness. You saw me… and you have always seen me. I always feel safe with you and for someone like me that is a gift of epic proportions. Thank you for socks, Tahitian pearls, counsel, lots of food, laughs, Vermont, Monster's Ball and beyonds. "You're the bomb boy, just keeping it real boo"…Thank you for being my best friend. Luv U

Achleigh-Ambur Gabrelle- "Harpo, I need you to come down here and hold this baby"… You have blossomed into quite an interestingly, funny, and independent young lady. Celebrate you every day Percy because you are worth celebrating! I love you Agent Sterling.

CL Freeman—You gifted me with the Secret and possibility. Thank you. I love you like corned beef and cabbage! You are the man, 1000 grand!

Chatone aka Tonald, you are one of the sweetest most giving people I know. Thank you for being you. Your love is so unconditional and true. My goodness. Big YAY! Love You Big Sis.

Appendix A

"Reproductive Medicine: Research Projects in Acupuncture -- Stener-Victorin 16 (2): 80 -- Acupuncture in Medicine." *Acupuncture in Medicine - BMJ Journals*. Elisabet Sterner-Victorian. Web. 27 Dec. 2011. <http://aim.bmj.com/content/16/2/80.abstract>.

Sterner-Victorin et al Acupuncture *Protocol for IVF*

Elisabet Stener-Victorin

Stener-Victorin et al Protocol

Eight treatments before retrieval

o

Treat the patient twice a week for four weeks up to retrieval

* Point Locations (all points are needled bilaterally)

o UB 23 (black clip) to UB 28 (red clip) (one lead)

o SP 6 (red clip) to UB 57 (black clip) (one lead)

o Electro-stimulation set from 0 – 100 Hz for 30 minutes

* TDP lamp on the low back is optional for the patient

* Needles

o 36 g 1-1 ½ inch needles

For full article: http://www.phoenixacupuncture.com/article1.html[/url]

Here is the Paulus (pre & post IVF acupuncture) protocol used in their research

Paulus et al. Protocol

* Treat 12-24 hours before embryo transfer

* Treat within 1 hour after embryo transfer

* Pre transfer points

o Du 20, PC 6, ST 29, SP 8, LIV 3

o Ear points

+ Rt. Shen, brain

+ Lt. Uterus,endocrine

* Place press tacks in each ear using the same points and ask patient to stimulate them during transfer.

* Post transfer points

o LI 4, SP 10, ST 36, SP 6

o Ear Points

+ Rt uterus, endocrine

+ Lt. Shen brain

+ Place press tacks in same pattern instruct patient to remove in 3 days

* Needles

o 32 g 1 ½ inch needles

o Stimulate to obtain deqi (Qi)

o Re-stimulate after 10 minutes, leave another 15 minutes Total Retention 25 minutes.

Appendix B

Wilson, J. H. "Viburnum Prunifolium, or Black Haw, in Abortion and Miscarriage." *Bmj*1.1318 (1886): 640-41. Print.

the complicated colon, and the presence of sacculi in that part of the canal.

The Ungulates.—Space will not permit the consideration of this family in any detail. So far as the alimentary canal can serve as a guide, it would appear certain that the ungulates take their descent from the rodents. The colic spiral and the colic loop reappear in a pronounced manner in the more specialised class of animal. The line of descent would appear to be in the following direction. From rodents with spirals (for example, the capybara) come the artiodactyla, the hogs coming first in the line of descent. From the hogs, the hippopotamide branch off and lead nowhere, and from the same trunk spring the ruminants. The colic spiral is carefully retained throughout, and the development of the ruminant stomach can be followed step by step. From rodents with loops spring the perissodactyla, the rhinoceros, the tapir, the horse, animals that all preserve the rodent outline of stomach, and accurately reproduce the colic loop.

ON PAPAIN AND ITS USE IN THE TREATMENT OF DYSPEPSIA.

By GEORGE HERSCHELL, M.D.Lond.,
Physician to the Farringdon General Dispensary.

For some time past, a drug has been before the medical world, called papain, which claims to be able to replace pepsin and pancreatin in medicine, but, for several reasons, has not come into general use. It is a powder, and is prepared from the juice of the *Carica papaia*, or melon-tree. There are at present two chief varieties of this drug on the market; namely, that sold by Christy, with which most of the experiments up to recently have been made, it having been before the profession some considerable time; and a papain quite lately introduced into this country, and prepared according to the process of Professor Finkler, who occupies the chair of physiology at the University of Bonn, and who for the last few years has been experimenting with the digestive ferments. This latter (papain, Finkler) is likely to prove of considerable use, as it is without the imperfections which have prevented papain (Christy) from doing so. In the first place, it is cheaper; in the second, it is less energetic. This we shall show to be a *sine quâ non.*

I will commence by an account of its properties as determined by Professor Finkler, which will advantageously compare with those of pepsin and pancreatin. 1. It digests equally in acid, alkaline, or neutral fluids, best of all in water. 2. It will dissolve 1,000 times its own weight of fresh blood-fibrin. 3. Its action is increased by the presence of pepsin and pancreatin. 4. It acts at the temperature of the body. 5. Meat infused with a solution of papain keeps, while undergoing a softening process, much longer than it does without it. From this, it can be inferred that it has an antiseptic as well as a peptonising action. 6. The product of its action is a pepton, which, from its properties, may be taken to be Meissner's *c* pepton. 7. Papain adheres to albumen to such a degree as to prevent its being removed by protracted washing with water. 8. Papain, in contrast to pepsin, acts when the resulting pepton-solution is highly concentrated. 9. The addition of antiseptics, such as salicylic or carbolic acids, does not interfere with its action. Hence, in papain (Finkler), we have apparently an ideal digestive ferment.

I will now pass on to consider the difference in properties of papain (Christy) and papain (Finkler). In experimenting with them, and comparing the results, it appears at first sight that the former is much more energetic than the latter; but, on further investigation, it will be seen that this apparent virtue really unfits it for internal use, inasmuch as, not content with converting the fibrin into pepton, it again splits it up into bodies soluble in alcohol, and analogous to leucin and tyrosin, which, so far from being of any use in digestion, are absolutely injurious. It is therefore evident that the chemical and medicinal results must be kept apart.

If .01 gramme of papain (Finkler) be placed with 10 grammes of fresh blood-fibrin, and 50cc. of water, at 45° to 50°C. (113 and 122 Fahr.), and put into an oven of the same temperature, the solution takes place in from forty-eight to eighty hours. If, on the other hand, papain (Christy), be used instead, in the same experiment, the solution takes place in a much shorter time. But here an important distinction comes in.

If to the result of each experiment be added 10 grammes of fresh blood-fibrin, it will be found that the papain (Finkler) will still dissolve this in twenty hours, while that containing the papain (Christy) will not dissolve at all. This proves that the former is a true catalytic ferment, and that the latter is not. An alcoholic extract of the latter

will also show the presence of the leucin and tyrosin-like bodies by the usual tests. These experiments are easy, and anyone can make them for himself without any very special apparatus.

Dr. Finkler states that he can prepare a papain identical in its action to that of Christy, by a different method. I have received a sample, and find it identical in its action with that of Christy. He has discarded this method in favour of that which he now uses, and which produces a papain, whose initial action is less energetic but is indefinitely prolonged. It is this papain (Finkler) which I have been for some time prescribing, and with which I have obtained very satisfactory results in cases of dyspepsia.

I find it chiefly valuable in the following classes of cases.

1. *Chronic Stomach-Catarrhs of Children.*—Everyone of us is familiar with that state in which we find children at times, and which is very frequently called "biliousness." It is characterised by loss of appetite, languor, pasty complexion, loss of sleep at night, and irritability during the day. There is frequently frontal headache, and the urine is loaded with lithates. If this state continue for any length of time the child emaciates, the unhealthy mucus which sheathes the stomach and intestines preventing the due absorption of the food. Cod-liver oil and compound syrup of the phosphates, which are generally given for this complaint as soon as the child begins to lose flesh, are not assimilated. Sometimes a cough develops, and the child is supposed to have incipient phthisis. I have found these cases rapidly improve with the following prescription:—℞ Papain (Finkler), gr. ½ - gr. j; sacch. lactis, gr. j; sodii bicarb., gr. v. M. To be taken after every meal. It is also advantageous to give a drop or two of tincture of nux vomica immediately before the meal in a little water. The papain probably acts by dissolving the mucus, and thus facilitating the absorption of the food.

2. *Acid Dyspepsia.*—This drug is extremely valuable in this form of indigestion. α. As it acts equally well in the presence of an alkali, a sufficient quantity of bicarbonate of soda may be given with it to neutralise the excess of acid in the stomach without impairing its peptonising power. b. Its antiseptic action checks the abnormal fermentation to which much of the accompanying flatulence is due. c. An antiseptic can be given with it to increase this action. I usually order it in the following manner:—℞ Papain (Finkler), gr. ij; sacch. lactis, gr. v. M. To be taken an hour after meals with the following draught:—℞ Sodii bicarb., gr. xv; glycerin. acid carbolic, ♏ viii; spirit. ammon. aromat., ♏ xx; aq. ad ʒiss. M. Fiat haustus. It appears that, taken one hour after a meal, a smaller dose of papain is required to produce the same result than if taken with the food.

3. *Cases where Severe Gastric Pain coming on Shortly after Eating is the Prominent Symptom.*—I have tried the drug upon twelve cases of this nature. Complete relief was given in ten, one case was partially relieved, and one completely failed to derive any benefit.

Apart from its internal use, papain will probably come into extensive use as a peptonising agent, to prepare ready digested food and enemata in the way in which pancreatin and pepsin are used at present.

VIBURNUM PRUNIFOLIUM, OR BLACK HAW, IN ABORTION AND MISCARRIAGE.

By JOHN HENRY WILSON, M.K.Q.C.P., M.R.C.S.E.,
Fellow of the Obstetrical Society; Consulting Physician-Accoucheur to the Ladies' Charity and Lying-in Hospital, Liverpool.

I am glad that the attention of the members of the British Medical Association has been drawn to the efficacy of this medicine in cases of abortion and miscarriage, by Dr. Macfie Campbell, and Dr. Leith Napier.

In the number of the *Liverpool Medico-Chirurgical Journal* for January, 1885, I reported six typical cases treated successfully by this medicine; and since then, after considerable experience, I have been more and more confirmed in its value. I cannot say it has always succeeded, but in those cases in which it failed, I have been able to account for its doing so. Either the medicine has not been commenced in time, and the ovum has been detached before the viburnum has been taken, or there has been some reason to suspect a syphilitic taint; and, in a case of fatty degeneration of the placenta, after not succeeding with the viburnum alone, chlorate of potash was taken in addition, with a good result.

Dr. Napier says, "some women abort on the slightest provocation," and they continue to do so, although every care may have been taken in the way of rest, medicine, etc., to prevent it. I have had many such cases, and have been greatly disappointed; but when I have had the opportunity of commencing the viburnum shortly before the antici-

April 3, 1886.]   THE BRITISH MEDICAL JOURNAL.   641

pated period, and continued it at intervals on the first appearance of threatening symptoms, these patients have invariably gone on to the full time, and done well, without being subjected to restrictions or debarred from active exercise.

In the next class of cases, where there may be reason to suspect even a partial separation of the ovum and a dilated external os, with severe pains and hemorrhage going on for hours, and the patient under the impression that she could not possibly go on to her full time, and when I had almost despaired of any benefit from the medicine, I have been astonished at its effect, more than three-fourths of these cases doing well.

The most sanguine advocate of viburnum could not expect it to do impossibilities, or to prevent abortion when there is "a gaping os, and a detached ovum presenting." One might as well expect to resuscitate a dead body by galvanism.

I have never seen ill consequences follow the administration of the medicine, however often the dose has been repeated. In two cases only has it been followed by slight headache. One patient inquired if she had not been taking quinine. The symptoms had been relieved; therefore it was not continued. In the other case, the patient had taken four grains of the extract every two hours. The only change was to extend the interval to four hours, and then gradually discontinue it.

Some patients have taken viburnum at intervals during the whole course of their pregnancy. It seems to act as an uterine tonic and sedative, and to relieve the woman of those harassing nervous forebodings which often lead to abortion. The patient, after taking only a few doses, has quite a changed expression. From a drawn, desponding look, her countenance becomes cheerful and happy.

Since I have prescribed viburnum, it has not been necessary to keep the women in the horizontal position more than a few days; whereas, under the old treatment, they occasionally spent weeks in bed, and, after all, abortion has taken place.

On some of the plantations in America, it is the popular belief a woman cannot abort if she be under the influence of black haw, although she may be taking medicine with a criminal intent. My experience would go far to confirm that opinion, for I have had patients in whom a succession of abortions have taken place, but, when under the influence of the medicine, they have been able to resist the severest tests—frights, falls, strains, etc.—and no ill effects have followed.

With regard to the mode of administering the drug: at first, the liquid extract was ordered, but the smell was so strong and objectionable, that the whole house became impregnated; and in two cases, where the stomach could not retain it, the liquid was given as an enema.

I now order the extract in pills of four grains, and find it a convenient form; as usually made, they soon absorb moisture, and run into a mass; but I now advise them gelatine-coated, as prepared by Parke, Davis, and Co., of Detroit, who seem to have been the first to introduce this medicine to the profession. I have no doubt others would make them equally well. These pills keep any length of time, and I advise my patients to keep a supply by them.

I have such confidence in viburnum prunifolium that I am anxious the profession should give it a trial, feeling assured they will not be disappointed.

OBSTETRIC MEMORANDA.

INVERSION OF UTERUS.

SHORTLY after leaving college, and while acting as assistant to a medical man, I was sent for hurriedly to attend a woman in her first confinement, and whom the messenger reported to be very ill; no medical man had been previously engaged. On my arrival I found that the child was born, and had been removed from the bed. On inspection of the patient, who was in a state of collapse, and meaning feebly, I saw, protruding from the vulva, what appeared to my inexperienced eye, like a fœtal head. Closer inspection, however, showed me that this was none other than the uterus, completely prolapsed and inverted, and with the placenta still attached. The amount of hæmorrhage was slight. I first carefully detached the placenta, and then, with the tips of my fingers, pressed back the uterus into the pelvic cavity, and had the satisfaction of replacing and reinverting the displaced organ. I then bound the woman up, and administered a stimulant; but she never rallied, and died a few hours later. In this case, the midwife acknowledged to me that the umbilical cord was pulled very forcibly; and, at the inquest subsequently held, the evidence seemed to show that the poor patient was rather roughly handled, and suffered a good deal subsequent to the birth of the child, and previous to my arrival.

In this case, the direct and immediate cause of the accident was the forcible traction of the umbilical cord by the midwife.
ROBERT F. SINCLAIR, M.B.
Belfast.

THERAPEUTIC MEMORANDA.

ERGOTIN IN THE TREATMENT OF PROFUSE HÆMOPTYSIS.

PROFESSOR BARTHOLOW, of Philadelphia, in reference to this question, says (*Practice of Medicine*, p. 378), "The most effective remedy is the hypodermatic injection of ergotin. Often the most severe bleeding will be at once arrested, when other means of treatment had been employed in vain." My own experience is quite in accord with this opinion; I know no remedy so reliable and so speedy in its action in severe cases. The following cases illustrate this action of ergotin.

CASE I.—A man, aged 30, in an advanced stage of pulmonary phthisis, with large cavities in both lungs, was seized with hæmoptysis, and lost a pint of blood in the three or four minutes which elapsed before I reached him. Five minutes after the hypodermic injection of 7 grains of ergotin, the bleeding had entirely ceased, and there was no recurrence of it for several days.

CASE II.—A man, aged 21, with phthisis affecting both lungs, but no decided evidence of excavation, seized with hæmoptysis, had lost more than 10 ounces of blood before the hypodermic injection of 4 grains of ergotin. After the injection, he brought up only two mouthfuls of blood, and then the hæmorrhage ceased entirely, and in half an hour he walked upstairs to bed, and there was no recurrence of the bleeding.

In both cases there was no sign of spontaneous arrest of the bleeding before the administration of ergotin, and I think the loss of blood would have been much greater before spontaneous arrest occurred. Cessation of bleeding after ergotin is more decided and abrupt than natural arrest; and in most cases the patient is ensured against further loss for some hours.   ROBERT ROBERTSON, M.D.,
Assistant-Physician to the Ventnor Consumption Hospital.

PHYSIOLOGICAL MEMORANDA.

THE VOICE A STRINGED INSTRUMENT.

THE question has often been discussed, as to what form of musical instrument the human voice most resembles. Many have regarded it as a form of reed-instrument; others have favoured the theory that it partakes of the nature of a wind-instrument; while some incline to the idea of a stringed instrument, such as the violin, or violoncello. With these latter I agree; and, as some observations I have lately made point in that direction, I take this opportunity of putting them on record. We have, I consider, reasons—anatomical, pathological, and what I will venture to call vocal—which confirm the "stringed-instrument theory."

Anatomical.—1. The vocal cords are two strings of yellow elastic tissue, capable of the most exact extension and relaxation. 2. They are covered with extremely fine and closely adherent mucous membrane, without any submucous tissue, and which is incapable of being thrown into wrinkles or folds, that would interfere with perfect vibration. 3. A muscle, the intrinsic tensor of the cords, the thyro-arytenoid, is attached in segments all along the vocal cords, and capable, by its contraction, of creating a state of tension of that part of the cord between the contracting filaments and the point of its insertion.

Pathological.—1. When the cords cannot approximate, from the interposition of mucus, tumours, etc., huskiness or loss of voice ensues; it is analogous to pressing the fiddle-string with the finger, without applying the bow. The aperture between the cords is too large to allow the air to be applied with sufficient force to produce the necessary vibrations, though the cords may be in an exact state of tension. 2. In inflammation (laryngitis) the aperture may remain normal; but the cords, owing to thickening, and the inflamed condition of the intrinsic muscles, are incapable of perfect tension. 3. In cases of paralysis of one cord, there is loss of volume or power, though weak notes can be correctly produced.

Vocal.—1. I have recently had the opportunity of examining the larynges of over fifty practised vocalists, and would venture to formulate the results of my observations in this way. High and low notes are produced through an unaltered vocal aperture, provided the

About the Author

"Your Truth is as unique as your fingerprints and you will never see what is truly possible for you, when you are looking through or walking in someone's truth..."

The World's #1 True Self Facilitator...

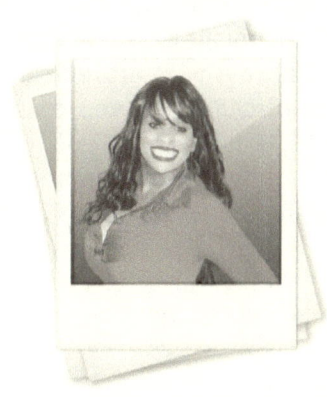

An in demand coach, trainer, author and speaker, Tiphanie "TK" Jamison VanDerLugt has cracked the code of traditional personal development, with her innovative process for creating immediate life-changing results by expanding what's truly possible for your life when you become a Self-Expert. Instead of positive thinking and affirmations, she is facilitating RADICAL Self EdYOUcation as the founder of The Yay Me University™- to women (+ cool men) around the world who are tired of failing and struggling to experience the life they desire (all of life's goodies) trying to be like everyone else and are finally ready to succeed, win, be happy and have wealth being their True Self. As the World's #1 True Self Facilitator, the guiding principle in all of her work, is, "…your truth is as unique as your fingerprints and the only path to true happiness, health, wealth, ease and infinite possibilities. Since possibilities create opportunities, how many opportunities will you miss, because someone else says it's not possible? You will never see what is possible for you, walking in or looking through someone else's truth." At The Yay Me University™, you are guided to discover your true self, so you boost your true wealth and live happily with days filled with YAY- the Easy Way.

Her book, "The Radical Self-Expert" was born out of her recognition that traditional personal development methods were not working and left her and countless others feeling like personal development misfits. Her method supercharges the discovery of your true self by playfully and powerfully inviting you to experience creating and generating a life and living that You LOVE, FREE from judgments and limitations, so you take bold actions + get rapid unprecedented results in any area of your life that isn't working as you desire it to. "Who would you be if you lost your ability to judge you... If you lost your ability to receive the judgments of others about you and make them your own?" asks, Tiphanie. She facilitates a one of a kind interactive RADICAL Self-Expert Experience virtually and in person to thrilled audiences around the world. Although it was not until her adulthood, that she welcomed her "misfit-ness", her commitment to "write your own rules, so you always win" attitude can be seen throughout her life. In the face of childhood abuse and neglect, she began college at the age of 15, taught college and university courses with no experience in her early 20's and opened a successful solo law practice with no training, mentors, or business experience.

Tiphanie developed and created 2 definitive laudable self-assessment tests: The True Self Test (also known as the True Self IQ Test) and The True To Self Test.

She has authored 3 books for print, The RADICAL Self-Expert, The Book on the True Self, The Book on the Pregnancy After Loss and the upcoming The Book on How to Pass the Bar.

Her formal education includes a Bachelors in Criminal Justice and Masters of Science in International Relations and a Juris Doctor; All of which she completed by the age of 27. For a copy of her academic credentials, please send your request to **Support@TheYayMe-University.com**. She is also a certified hypnotist, meditation master and nlp certified practitioner.

Tiphanie is a licensed attorney for the 9th Federal District and the State of California.

A bit quirky and more tomboy than she appears, Tiphanie's profound intellect and vibrancy, make for an adventurous and imaginative environment, in which self-growth is more delightful than difficult. She is a fun, passionate, sports jock who celebrates her feminine curves, and loves soft rock music from the 70s and 80s.

Endnotes

i   Gurevich, Rachel. "Clomid - All About Clomid." *Fertility - Infertility - Getting Pregnant - Fertility Treatments - Coping With Infertility*. About.com, 11 Nov. 2011. Web. 16 Dec. 2011. <http://infertility.about.com/od/infertilitytreatments/a/clomid101.htm>.

ii   Dr. Bruce Lipton Ph.D. and author of "The Biology Of Belief" –*Keynote speaker at the 2005 International BodyTalk Association Member Conference.

iii   Lipton, Bruce H. *The Biology of Belief: Unleashing the Power of Consciousness, Matter, and Miracles*. Carlsbad, CA: Hay House, 2008. Print.

iv   "Bacterial Vaginosis." *Wikipedia*. Wikimedia Foundation, 08 Feb. 2013. Web. 08 Feb. 2013.

v   The products and information (individually and collectively "The Materials") obtained through this website, including but not limited to personal consultations and from The Yay Me University, are for informational purposes only and are not intended to replace or substitute any advice from your medical practitioner, a qualified doctor, or any other professional and advisor. You should consult a qualified health practitioner before implementing any of the suggestions found on The Website, and should not give up any medical treatment you are using without the express consent of a medical professional.

The Materials obtained through The Website cannot serve as a substitute for face-to-face professional advice and are not intended to diagnose or treat any illness, metabolic disorder, disease or health problem. Always consult your physician or health care provider before beginning any nutrition or exercise program or using The Materials obtained through The Website. You voluntarily undertake your use of The Materials contained on The Website, and you assume all risk and responsibility for any such use, including but not limited to any increase in severity of your infertility condition. The Materials found on The Website may not be suitable for your own personal circumstances, you may not receive any benefit from use of The Materials, and The Website does not guarantee that you will achieve any specific result.

---

* These statements have not been evaluated by the Food and Drug Administration. This product is not intended to diagnose, treat, cure or prevent any disease. If you are pregnant, nursing, taking medication, or have a medical condition, consult your physician before using this product.

The Website is neither responsible nor liable for injury resulting from the use, misuse, and/or abuse of The Materials. You hereby release and agree to hold harmless The Website, its directors, officers, employees, agents, representatives, successors, advisors, consultants, and assigns from any and all causes of action and claims of any nature resulting from your use of The Materials.

The content and information accessed through The Website represents the content and information as at the date of publication. As conditions change, The Website reserves the right to alter and update the content to reflect the new conditions.

The Website does not assume any responsibility for errors, inaccuracies or omissions in any of the articles or information posted on the website. The website content may contain inaccuracies or typographical errors. This website may contain certain historical information. Historical information necessarily is not current and is provided for your reference only. Further, The Website is not responsible if information that is made available on this website is not accurate, reliable, complete, timely, or current. Any reliance upon the material on this website will be at your own risk. The Website reserves the right to modify the contents of the website at any time, but The Website has no obligation to update any information on this website. You agree that it is your responsibility to monitor changes to the website.

Tiphanie Jamison VanDerLugt, TheRadicalSelfExpert.com, The RADICAL Self ExpertMethod.com ,TheBookonPregnancyAfterLoss.com, and any and all sites related to, owned and/or administrated by, including but not limited to ITS OWNERS, ITS AFFILIATES, AND ITS SPONSORS ARE NEITHER RESPONSIBLE NOR LIABLE FOR ANY DIRECT, INDIRECT, INCIDENTAL, CONSEQUENTIAL, SPECIAL, EXEMPLARY, PUNITIVE OR OTHER DAMAGES ARISING OUT OF OR RELATING IN ANY WAY TO THE SITE, SITE-RELATED SERVICES AND/OR CONTENT OR INFORMATION CONTAINED WITHIN THE SITE. YOUR SOLE REMEDY FOR DISSATISFACTION WITH THE SITE AND/OR SITE-RELATED SERVICES IS TO STOP USING THE SITE AND/OR THOSE SERVICES.

Disclaimer: The information on The Book on Pregnancy After Loss and all associated sites with Tiphanie , Jamison VanDerLugt is provided for educational purposes only and is not intended to treat, diagnose or prevent any disease. The entire contents of this website are based upon the opinions of Tiphanie Jamison VanDerLugt, unless otherwise noted. Individual articles are based upon the opinions of the respective author, who retains copyright as marked. The information on this website is not intended to replace a one-on-one relationship with a qualified health care professional and is not intended as medical advice. It is intended as a sharing of knowledge and information from the research and experience of Tiphanie Jamison VanDerLugt and her community. We encourage you to make your own health care decisions based upon your research and in partnership with a qualified health care professional.

vi   Kevin Hogan, www.KevinHogan.com,

vii   Hill, Napoleon. *Think and Grow Rich*. Meriden, CT: Ralston Society, 1939. Print.

viii Master Key System, Charles Haanel, Part VII

ix   Agarwal A et al. Effect of cell phone usage on semen analysis in men attend-
      ing infertility clinic: An observational study. Fertility and Sterility January 2008;
      89:124.

x   "Reproductive Medicine: Research Projects in Acupuncture -- Stener-Victorin
      16 (2): 80 -- Acupuncture in Medicine." *Acupuncture in Medicine - BMJ Jour-
      nals*. Elisabet Sterner-Victorian. Web. 27 Dec. 2011. <http://aim.bmj.com/con-
      tent/16/2/80.abstract>.

xi   Null, Gary, and Amy McDonald. *Get Healthy Now! with Gary Null: a Complete
      Guide to Prevention, Treatment, and Healthy Living*. New York: Seven Stories,
      2001.

xii

xiii Tempfer, C., C. Kurz, E. Bentz, G. Unfried, K. Walch, U. Czizek, and J. Huber. "A
      Combination Treatment of Prednisone, Aspirin, Folate, and Progesterone in
      Women with Idiopathic Recurrent Miscarriage: a Matched-pair Study." *Fertility
      and Sterility*86.1 (2006): 145-48. Print.

xiv   According to David Hoffman "No side effects or drug interactions have been
      reported."2

      Fred J Petersen (1905) Petersen's Materia Medica. Self-published. pp 141 - 142.

      David Hoffman (2003) Medical Herbalism - The science and practice of herbal medi-
      cine. Healing Arts Press. pp. 594

      Michael Castleman (1991). The Healing Herbs. Rodale Press. pp. 79–81.

xv   Petersen, 1905.

xvi   Wilson, J. H. "Viburnum Prunifolium, or Black Haw, in Abortion and Miscar-
      riage." *Bmj*1.1318 (1886): 640-41. Print.

xvii Id.

xviii

xix   Brown, Royden. "Bee Pollen: The Perfect Food." *Http://arthritistrust.org*.
      Web.<http://arthritistrust.org/Articles/Bee%20Pollen%20The%20Perfect%20
      Food.pdf>. "Bee Bread." *Wikipedia, the Free Encyclopedia*. Web. 27 Dec. 2011.
      <http://en.wikipedia.org/wiki/Bee_pollen>. Townsend, Gordan F., and Colin C.
      Lucas. "The Chemical Nature of Royal Jelly." Web. <http://www.ncbi.nlm.nih.
      gov/pmc/articles/PMC1265395/?page=1>. Lewis, Randine A. *The Infertility Cure:
      the Ancient Chinese Wellness Program for Getting Pregnant and Having Healthy
      Babies*. Boston, MA: Little, Brown, 2005. Print.

xx   "Take Folic Acid before Youâ™re Pregnant | Pregnancy | March of Dimes." *Preg-
      nancy, Baby, Prematurity, Birth Defects | March of Dimes*. Web. <http://www.mar-
      chofdimes.com/pregnancy/folicacid_before.html>.

xxi Henmi H et al. Effects of ascorbic acid supplementation on serum progesterone levels in patients with a luteal phase defect. Fertility and Sterility August 2003; 80:459-461.

xxii

xiii Lewis, Randine. "Male Infertility (improving Sperm Quality) - Vancouver BC (British Columbia) Canada - Acupuncture and Traditional Chinese Medicine for Infertility, Spence Pentland Acupuncturist, Fertility Clinic, IVF (in Vitro Fertilization), IUI (inta Uterine Insemination) , Other Artificial Reproductive Technology, and Natural Conception, Fertility Diet Nutrition, Sex, Fertility Awareness Methods, Reproductive Anatomy Physiology, Lifestyle, Herbs Impotence, Low Sex Drive, Stress." *Infertility & IVF Vancouver BC (BC (British Columbia)) Canada - Acupuncture and Traditional Chinese Medicine for Infertility, Spence Pentland Acupuncturist and Practitioner of Chinese Medicine, IVF (in Vitro Fertilization), IUI (inta Uterine Insemination) , Other Artificial Reproductive Technology, and Natural Conception, Fertility Diet Nutrition, Sex, Fertility Awareness Methods, Reproductive Anatomy Physiology, Lifestyle, Herbs.* Web. 27 Dec. 2011. <http://infertility.health-info.org/male-infertility/male-infertility-improve-sperm-quality.html>.

xxiv Roseff SJ. Improvement in sperm quality and function with French maritime pine tree bark extract. J Reprod Med. 2002 Oct;47(10):821-4. PMID: 12418064

xxv Id.

xxvi Garolla, A., M. Maiorino, A. Roverato, A. Roveri, F. Ursini, and C. Foresta. "Oral Carnitine Supplementation Increases Sperm Motility in Asthenozoospermic Men with Normal Sperm Phospholipid Hydroperoxide Glutathione Peroxidase Levels." Fertility and Sterility 83.2 (2005): 355-61. Print.

xxvii

xxviii Moriyama, H., K. Nakamura, N. Sanda, E. Fujiwara, S. Seko, A. Yamazaki, M. Mizutani, K. Sagami, and T. Kitano. "Studies on the Usefulness of a Long-term, High-dose Treatment of Methylcobalamin in Patients with Oligozoospermia." Hinyokika Kiya 33.1 (1987): 151-6. Print.

xxix Wong, W., et al., "Effects of folic acid and zinc sulfate on male factor subfertility: a double-blind, randomized, placebo-controlled trial," Fertility and Sterility, Vol. 77, No.3, March 2002.

xxx Tikkiwal M et al. Effect of zinc administration on seminal zinc and fertility of oligospermic males. Ind J Phys Pharm 1987; 31:30-34.

xxxi Colagar AH, Marzony ET, Chaichi MJ. Zinc levels in seminal plasma are associated with sperm quality in fertile and infertile men. Nutr. Res. 2009 Feb; 29(2):82-8

xxxii Piomboni, Paola, Laura Gambera, Francesca Serafini, Giovanna Campanella, Giuseppe Morgante, and Vincenzo De Leo. "Sperm Quality Improvement after Natural Anti-oxidant Treatment of Asthenoteratospermic Men with Leukocytospermia." Asian Journal of Andrology 10.2 (2008): 201-06. Print.

Vicari, E. Effectiveness of a short-term anti-oxidative high-dose therapy on IVF program outcome in infertile male patients with previous excessive sperm Radical Oxygen Species production, persistent even following antimicrobials administered for epididymitis: preliminary results. In Ambrosini, A., Melis, G.B., Dalla Pria, S. and Dessole, S. (eds), Int. Meeting on Infertility and Assisted Reproductive Technology (From Research to Therapy), Porto Cervo, June 11–14, 1997. Monduzzi, Ed, International Proceedings Division, Bologna, Italy, pp. 93–97.

[xxxiii] "Antioxidant Blend for Male Fertility and Sperm Health." *FertilAid Fertility Supplements for Women & Men*. Web. <http://www.fertilaid.com/antioxidant-blend.asp>.

[xxxiv] Keskes-Ammar, L., N. Feki-Chakroun, T. Rebai, Z. Sahnoun, H. Ghozzi, S. Hammami, K. Zghal, H. Fki, J. Damak, and A. Bahloul. "Sperm Oxidative Stress And The Effect Of An Oral Vitamin E And Selenium Supplement On Semen Quality In Infertile Men."*Archives of Andrology* 49.2 (2003): 83-94. Print.

[xxxv] Akmal, Mohammed, J.Q. Qadri, Noori S. Al-Waili, Shahiya Thangal, Afrozul Haq, and Khelod Y. Saloom. "Improvement in Human Semen Quality After Oral Supplementation of Vitamin C." Journal of Medicinal Food 9.3 (2006): 440-42. Print.

[xxxvi] "Vitamin D Is Positively Associated with Sperm Motility and Increases Intracellular Calcium in Human Spermatozoa." Oxford Journal. Print.

[xxxvii] Thys-Jacobs S, Starkey P, Bernstein D, Tian J. Calcium carbonate and the premenstrual syndrome: effects on premenstrual and menstrual symptoms. Premenstrual Syndrome Study Group. Am J Obstet Gynecol 1998;179:444-52.

Wai Yee Wong, Gert Flik, Pascal M.W. Groenen, Dorine W. Swinkels, chris M.G. Thomas, Jenny H.J. Copius-Peereboom, Hans M.W.M Merkus and Regine P.M. Steegers-Theunissen. The impact of calcium, magnesium, zinc, and copper in blood and seminal plasma on semen parameters in men. Reproductive Toxicity Vol 15, Issue 2, March 2001, Pages 131-136.

Thys-Jacobs S, Ceccarelli S, Bierman A, Weisman H, Cohen MA, Alvir J. Calcium supplementation in premenstrual syndrome: a randomized crossover trial. J Gen Intern Med. 1989 May-Jun; 4 (3): 183-9.

[xxxviii] Wai Yee Wong, Gert Flik, Pascal M.W. Groenen, Dorine W. Swinkels, Chris M.G. Thomas, Jenny H.J. Copius-Peereboom, Hans M.W.M Merkus and Regine P.M. Steegers-Theunissen. The impact of calcium, magnesium, zinc, and copper in blood and seminal plasma on semen parameters in men. Reproductive Toxicity Vol 15, Issue 2, March 2001, Pages 131-136.

www.ingramcontent.com/pod-product-compliance
Lightning Source LLC
Chambersburg PA
CBHW020541290526
45786CB00002B/989